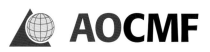

Kenneth E Fleisher | Risto Kontio | Sven Otto

Antiresorptive Drug-related Osteonecrosis of the Jaw (ARONJ)—a Guide to Research

Preface

The advances in medicine and surgery over the past several decades have reached a new phase: the science of bone and its manipulation has evolved concurrently. The nature of bone pathology has also changed. As the incidence of osteoradionecrosis over the past several years has decreased, the treatment of bone with antiosteoclastic drugs for prevention of bone loss and control of metastasis has produced new dilemmas and serious unpredictable implications. Antiosteoclastic drugs have now been associated with an increasing epidemic of osteonecrosis of the jaw.

Osteonecrosis of the jaw (ONJ) is defined as exposed alveolar or palatal bone where oral mucosa is normally found and that has broken out in the absence of previous radiotherapy to the jaw, is not a metastatic lesion, and has not healed within 8 weeks. The pathogenesis of ONJ is most likely multifactorial. Consideration of major risk factors associated with ONJ may provide insight into possible pathogenic mechanisms. There is a strong association of ONJ with suppression of bone turnover and the magnitude and duration of antiosteoclastic drug exposure appears to significantly affect the risk. Whether ONJ is associated with, induced by, or related to antiosteoclastic drugs is one of the several open issues.

Local factors in the mouth clearly play a role in determining risk. Traumatic events to oral mucosa, such as injury from poorly fitting dentures, results in exposure of bone and microbial flora increasing bone remodelling.

Since the original description of bisphosphonate-related ONJ in 2003, awareness of the condition has increased and medical management has evolved from an initially conservative, less interventional approach to a more aggressive surgical approach recently. Sensitive image technology with novel fluorescence techniques among others have continued to advance the diagnosis and management of ONJ. As the understanding of ONJ management and outcomes is progressing, further evaluation of the natural history of ONJ is warranted.

After the previously successful clinical priority program (CPP) "Imaging and Planning in Surgery", the AOCMF Research and Development Commission approved a subsequent CPP: "Antiosteoclastic drugs and their impact on maxillofacial surgery– diagnosis, prevention, surgery, and treatment modalities (ARONJ)" in 2014. Over the past 2 years, the commission has issued three calls for grant applications in this clinically important focus field. This book "Antiresorptive Drug-related Osteonecrosis of the Jaw (ARONJ)—a Guide to Research" has evolved and received the present structure and topics as a result of discussion, review, and coordination between the book editors Kenneth Fleisher, Risto Kontio, and Sven Otto. The book was initiated to launch up-to-date scientific data about the nature of ARONJ, its pathogenesis, diagnosis, and treatment, but above all, tries to bring to light what is known about this complex disease. We hope that through this book we can share this knowledge with the reader.

Some of the authors have been involved with AOCMF education for years, while others have not previously participated in AOCMF or AO Foundation activities but are recognized internationally as experts and researchers in this topic. We are most grateful to all the authors, who took time out from their busy lives to contribute and provide the latest information on ARONJ as it relates to current and future research. They are responsible for the success of this book.

We offer our sincere thanks to AOCMF R&D Commission members, Dan Buchbinder, Ed Ellis, Sabine Girod, Riitta Seppanen, and Warren Schubert. The commission approved and participated with great enthusiasm in the project.

Our special thanks go to Ms Anita Anthon and Ms Mirjam Bucher, who tirelessly coordinated the project, organized the meetings, and enabled the planning in making this book. Our thanks also to AO Education Institute for their assistance with design and production.

Kenneth E Fleisher
Risto Kontio
Sven Otto

Contributors

Editors

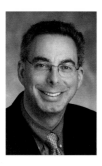

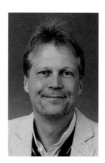

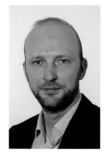

Kenneth E Fleisher, DDS, FAAOMS
Clinical Associate Professor
Department of Oral and Maxillofacial Surgery
New York University College of Dentistry
New York University Langone
Medical Center and Bellevue Hospital Center
New York, USA

Risto Kontio, MD, DDS, PhD
Docent, Senior Maxillofacial Surgeon
Chair, Department of OMFS
Helsinki University Hospital
Chair, R&D Commission AOCMF
Kasarminkatu 11-13
00029 HUS Helsinki, Finland

Sven Otto, MD, DDS, FEBOMFS
Senior Consultant
Department of Oral and Maxillofacial Surgery
Ludwig Maximilians University of Munich
Munich, Germany

Authors

Matthew R Allen, PhD
IU School of Medicine
Department of Anatomy & Cell Biology
635 Barnhill Drive MS 5045P
Indianapolis, USA 46202

Niloufar Amintavakoli, DDS, MSc
Clinical Assistant Professor
Department of Oral and Maxillofacial Pathology,
Radiology, and Medicine New York University
New York, USA

Alberto Bedogni, MD, FEBOMS
Department of Neurosciences-DNS
Unit of Maxillofacial Surgery
University of Padua
Via Giustiniani 2
I-35128 Padua, Italy

James L Borke, PhD
Professor
Assistant Dean for Biomedical Sciences
College of Dental Medicine
Western University of Health Sciences
309 E, Second Street
Pomona, USA 91766-1854

King Chong Chan, DMD, MS
Clinical Assistant Professor
Department of Oral and Maxillofacial Pathology,
Radiology, and Medicine
New York University College of Dentistry
New York, USA

Ezher H Dayisoylu, DDS
Faculty of Dentistry
Department of Oral and Maxillofacial Surgery
Karadeniz Technical University
Trabzon, Turkey

Stefano Fedele, DDS, PhD
University College London
UCL Eastman Dental Institute
NIHR University College London Hospitals
Biomedical Research Centre
London, United Kingdom

Kenneth E Fleisher, DDS, FAAOMS
Clinical Associate Professor
Department of Oral and Maxillofacial Surgery
New York University College of Dentistry
New York University Langone Medical Center and
Bellevue Hospital Center
New York, USA

Riham Fliefel, DDS
Department of Oral and Maxillofacial Surgery
Alexandria University
Alexandria, Egypt
Department of Experimental Surgery and Regenerative Medicine
Ludwig-Maximilians-University of Munich
Munich, Germany

Bente Brokstad Herlofson, DDS, Dr Odont
Associate Professor
Oral and Maxillofacial Surgeon
Department of Oral Surgery and Oral Medicine
Faculty of Dentistry
University of Oslo
Oslo, Norway

Risto Kontio, MD, DDS, PhD
Docent, Senior Maxillofacial Surgeon
Chair, Department of OMFS
Helsinki University Hospital
Chair, R&D Commission AOCMF
Kasarminkatu 11-13
00029 HUS Helsinki, Finland

Tae-Geon Kwon, DDS, PhD
Professor
Department of Oral & Maxillofacial Surgery
Kyungpook National University
Daegu, Korea

Robert E Marx, DDS
Professor of Surgery and Chief
University of Miami Miller School of Medicine
Division of Oral and Maxillofacial Surgery
9380 SW 150 Street, Suite 170
Miami, USA 33176

Sven Otto, MD, DDS, FEBOMFS
Senior Consultant
Department of Oral and Maxillofacial Surgery
Ludwig-Maximilians-University of Munich
Munich, Germany

Christoph Pautke, MD, DMD
Medizin and Ästhetik
Clinic for Oral and Maxillofacal Surgery
Lenbachplatz 2a
80333 Munich, Germany
Department of Oral and Maxillofacial Surgery
University of Munich
Lindwurmstr. 2a
80337 Munich, Germany

Oliver Ristow, MD, DDS
Department of Oral and Maxillofacial Surgery
University of Heidelberg
Im Neuenheimer Feld 400
D-69120 Heidelberg, Germany

Morten Schiodt, DDS, Dr Odont
Senior Maxillofacial Consultant
Department of Oral & Maxillofacial Surgery
Copenhagen University Hospital
Copenhagen, Denmark

Pit J Voss, MD, DMD
Department of Oral and Maxillofacial Surgery
University of Freiburg
Hugstetter Str 55
79106 Freiburg, Germany

Stephan Zeiter, PhD
Senior Project Leader
AO Research Institute
Clavadelerstrasse 8
7270 Davos, Switzerland

Table of contents

1 Definition, nomenclature, and classification of antiresorptive drug-related osteonecrosis of the jaw (ARONJ)

Tae-Geon Kwon

1 Introductory questions

In this opening chapter, the following questions are raised and discussed:

- When was bone necrosis first reported and how is it defined?
- What definitions for antiresorptive drug-related osteonecrosis of the jaw (ARONJ) exist?
- Why are different terms used and why are there so many?
- How is ARONJ classified?

2 Definition

According to a review article by Nixon in 1983 [1], bony necrosis was first described by a Professor James Russell in 1794, and the possibility of osteonecrosis due to an aseptic condition was first proposed in the early 20th century. Until recently, osteonecrosis had been considered synonymous with avascular necrosis or aseptic necrosis, which is frequently encountered in femoral head necrosis or radiation-induced necrosis of the jaw. Therefore, osteonecrosis had usually been regarded as a necrosis of bone caused by obstruction of the blood supply.

The initial reports of osteonecrosis of the jaw (ONJ) after bisphosphonate (BP) administration designated this condition as "avascular necrosis of the jaw" [2] or "avascular bone necrosis" [3] due to the similarities of the clinical manifestation of ONJ caused by radiation therapy and exposure to BPs, including the presence of nonvital and exposed bone with loss of the overlying mucosa. Consequently, the definition of ONJ after radiation therapy (osteoradionecrosis) had been similarly applied to ONJ after BP administration. Osteoradionecrosis is defined as exposed irradiated bone that fails to recover within 3 months in the absence of a residual or recurrent tumor [4]. A period of 3 months was considered because simple radionecrosis can spontaneously heal within a short period of time. Several authors have

suggested that the period of bone exposure required to meet the definition of osteoradionecrosis should be at least 2 months [5, 6] or longer than 6 months [7].

The working definition of ONJ after BP treatment was first proposed by an Australian consensus guideline as "an area of exposed bone that persists for more than 6 weeks" [8. 9]. A 2007 position paper from the American Association of Oral and Maxillofacial Surgeons (AAOMS) defined bisphosphonate-related osteonecrosis of the jaw (BRONJ) [10]. The diagnosis of BRONJ is made if all three of the following characteristics are present: 1) Current or previous treatment with a BP; 2) Exposed necrotic bone in the maxillofacial region that had persisted for more than 8 weeks; 3) No history of radiation therapy to the jaws. There is no scientific explanation as to why the duration of bone exposure should be more than 8 weeks, however, it was assumed that an 8-week healing period would be sufficient for most infectious and inflammatory jaw lesions to heal normally even though postoperative infection or systemic disease was present [11]. A Canadian consensus guideline emphasized the 8-week period of clinical observation because exposed bone should be followed-up to confirm whether the soft tissues would heal spontaneously [12]. In its 2009 position paper, the AAOMS removed the term "necrotic" from the definition of BRONJ and established "stage 0" (early stage) for this disease. Aside from this change, the definition of BRONJ given by the 2009 AAOMS guideline was nearly the same as that given in 2007 [13].

The recent definition from the 2014 AAOMS position paper included significant modifications compared to the 2009 position paper [14]. Under the 2014 definition, the following characteristics were defined: 1) Current or previous treatment with antiresorptive or antiangiogenic agents; 2) Exposed bone or bone that can be probed through an intraoral or extraoral fistula(e) in the maxillofacial region that has persisted for more than 8 weeks; 3) No history of radiation therapy to the jaws or obvious metastatic disease of the jaws. The previous description of ONJ as "exposed necrotic bone" was changed to "exposed bone or bone that can be probed through an intraoral or extraoral fistula". This is an important change to the definition of ONJ. However, there are limitations in these definitions because ONJ is not a histologically proven term and relies on only one clinical finding and two types of anamnestic information. A list of the changes to the definition of ONJ after BP administration is shown in **Table 1-1**.

3   Nomenclature

Osteoradionecrosis has also been frequently referred to as "osteomyelitis of irradiated bone", "osteonecrosis", "radioosteomyelitis", or "septic osteoradionecrosis". Like osteoradionecrosis, BRONJ has also been defined using a variety of terms, including "bisphosphonate-induced osteonecrosis of the jaw (BIONJ)" [15, 16] and "bisphosphonate-associated osteonecrosis of the jaw (BAONJ)" [12, 17, 18]. Some authors have emphasized the infectious cause of ONJ and used the term "bisphosphonate-associated osteomyelitis of the jaw (BAOMJ)" [19] or "bisphosphonate-related osteomyelitis of the jaw (BROMJ)" [20].

The term "associated" implies that a specific factor is assumed to be the cause of the disease whereas "related" implies that a specific factor was confirmed to be the cause of the disease [21]. The term "induced" implies a more direct cause-effect relationship; it is variously used based on the clinician's perception of the degree of proof that the BP is the cause of the jaw necrosis.

The terms for BRONJ, BAONJ, BIONJ, DIONJ, and MRONJ have recently been consolidated by the term antiresorptive drug-related osteonecrosis of the jaw (ARONJ) because of clinical reports of osteonecrosis of the jaw related to non BP antiresorptive medications such as denosumab or cathepsin K inhibitors [22]. However, there is some argument regarding this terminology due to the fundamental differences in the pharmacodynamics and accumulative toxicity of BPs and denosumab. Therefore, those authors argued that these two disease entities cannot be categorized as a single ONJ [23]. Another article used the term "denosumab-related osteonecrosis of the jaw, DRONJ" to differentiate the disease condition of BRONJ [24, 25]. To additionally include the antiangiogenic agents such as sunitinib or bevacizumab (vascular endothelial growth factor (VEGF) pathway inhibitor) to antiresorptive drugs, "drug-related osteonecrosis of the jaw, DRONJ" had been suggested [26]. In 2014, the AAOMS position paper also changed the term from BRONJ to medication-related osteonecrosis of the jaw (MRONJ), reflecting the potential risk of osteonecrosis associated with antiresorptive (denosumab) and antiangiogenic therapies [14]. In 2015, the International Task Force on Osteonecrosis of the Jaw also defined BP and denosumab as antiresorptive agents [27]. In this chapter, and throughout this publication, we use the term "antiresorptive drug-related osteonecrosis of the jaw (ARONJ)" based on the confirmed relationship between antiresorptive drugs and ONJ.

Only a limited number of cases of ONJ after administration of denosumab or antiangiogenic agents have been described, and the terminology of the disease may still be changed or modified if the pathophysiological mechanism is more clearly understood in the future.

Year	Definition	Endorsed by
2006	**Position paper** [8] Bisphosphonate and osteonecrosis of the jaw (ONJ) Working definition of ONJ: an area of exposed bone that persists for more than 6 weeks	Australian and New Zealand Bone and Mineral Society, Osteoporosis Australia, Medical Oncology Group of Australia, and the Australian Dental Association
2007	**2007 AAOMS position paper** [10] Bisphosphonate-related osteonecrosis of the jaw (BRONJ), if each of the following three characteristics are present: 1. Current or previous treatment with a BP 2. Exposed, necrotic bone in the maxillofacial region that has persisted for more than 8 weeks 3. No history of radiation therapy to the jaws	American Association of Oral and Maxillofacial Surgeons
2007	**Report of the Task Force of the ASBMR** [18] Bisphosphonate-associated osteonecrosis of the jaw (ONJ) 1. Confirmed case: defined as an area of exposed bone in the maxillofacial region that did not heal within 8 weeks after identification by a health care provider, in a patient that was receiving or had been exposed to a BP and had not had radiation therapy to the craniofacial region 2. Suspected case: defined as an area of exposed bone in the maxillofacial region that had been identified by a health care provider and had been present for <8 weeks in a patient that was receiving or had been exposed to a BP and had not had radiation therapy to the craniofacial region	American Society for Bone and Mineral Research
2008	**Canadian Consensus Practice Guidelines** [12] Bisphosphonate-associated ONJ Clinically in the presence of exposed bone in the maxillofacial region for more than 8 weeks in the absence of radiotherapy to the jaw. (If the exposed bone has been present for less than 8 weeks, it should be followed to confirm that soft tissues close; such a case would be described as a suspected case of osteonecrosis)	Canadian Association of Oral and Maxillofacial Surgeons, Canadian Society of Endocrinology and Metabolism, Canadian Academy of Oral and Maxillofacial Pathology and Oral Medicine, American Association of Clinical Endocrinologists, International Bone and Mineral Society, International Society of Clinical Densitometry
2009	**2009 AAOMS position paper** [13] BRONJ 1. Current or previous treatment with a BP 2. Exposed bone in the maxillofacial region that has persisted for more than 8 weeks 3. No history of radiation therapy to the jaws	American Association of Oral and Maxillofacial Surgeons
2010	**Position paper from the Allied Task Force Committee, Japan** [28] Bisphosphonate-related osteonecrosis of the jaw Adopts the definition and diagnostic criteria for BRONJ as stated by the 2009 AAOMS position paper	Japanese Society for Bone and Mineral Research, Japan Osteoporosis Society, Japanese Society of Periodontology, Japanese Society for Oral and Maxillofacial Radiology, Japanese Society of Oral and Maxillofacial Surgeons
2011	**Executive summary of recommendations from the American Dental Association Council on Scientific Affairs** [22] Antiresorptive agent-induced ONJ (ARONJ) Adopted the definition and diagnostic criteria for BRONJ as stated by the 2009 AAOMS position paper but extended criteria to encompass cases associated with the use of any antiresorptive agents	American Dental Association Council on Scientific Affairs
2014	**2014 AAOMS position paper** [14] Medication-related osteonecrosis of the jaw (MRONJ), if each of the following three characteristics are present: 1. Current or previous treatment with antiresorptive or antiangiogenic agents 2. Exposed bone or bone that can be probed through an intraoral or extraoral fistula(e) in the maxillofacial region that has persisted for more than 8 weeks 3. No history of radiation therapy to the jaws or obvious metastatic disease of the jaws	American Association of Oral and Maxillofacial Surgeons
2015	**Diagnosis and Management of Osteonecrosis of the Jaw: A Systematic Review and International Consensus** [27] Osteonecrosis of the jaw 1. Exposed bone in the maxillofacial region that does not heal within 8 weeks after identification by a health care provider 2. Exposure to an antiresorptive agent 3. No history of radiation therapy to the craniofacial region	International Task Force on Osteonecrosis of the Jaw

Table 1-1 Definitions of osteonecrosis of the jaw after administration of bisphosphonate and antiresorptive agents.

4   Classification

In the 2007 AAOMS position paper, BRONJ was classified in detail according to the severity of the clinical findings [10]. In particular, patients with soft tissue dehiscence and bone exposure were regarded as having established BRONJ. Established BRONJ without infection was regarded as stage 1. Stages 2 and 3 were categorized according to the severity of the infection and secondary complications such as pathologic fracture (**Fig 1-1**). Interestingly, a report from a task force of the American Society for Bone and Mineral Research (2007) did not provide a classification system according to the severity of BRONJ [18]. The Canadian consensus guideline (2008) classified BRONJ into stages 1, 2, and 3, similar to the 2007 AAOMS paper [12]. However, there was no "at risk" category in their classification. They

emphasized differential diagnosis based on spontaneous sequestration with ulceration of the lingual mandibular torus, which is self-limiting within 3 days to 12 weeks. In 2009, the revised AAOMS position paper added a new category, "stage 0", to "include patients with nonspecific symptoms or clinical and radiographic abnormalities that might have been due to BP exposure". The unknown potential risk that stage 0 could develop into a higher stage was considered. At the same time, the definition of stage 3 was also modified to include various degrees of bone destruction in the maxilla and mandible [13]. However, this classification system has been criticized in relation to whether direct exposure of the bone is a prerequisite for the diagnosis of ARONJ. Stage 0, with minimal bone exposure with sinus tract, sometimes accompanies a large necrotic sequestrum and can develop into higher stages [26, 29, 30]. The most

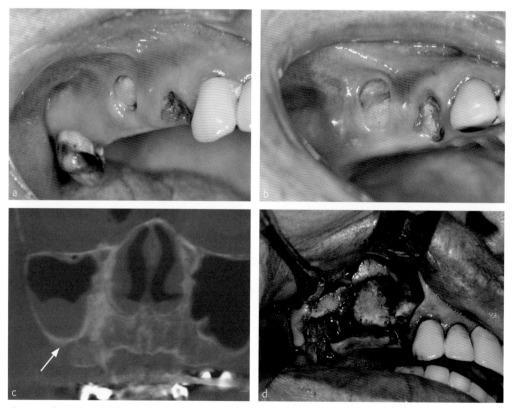

Fig 1-1a–d   Patients with 3 years of previous alendronate treatment showed exposed bone without evidence of infection or inflammation (stage 1), as with this patient (**a**). At 3 months after the initial diagnosis, patients developed a dull pain and infection in the exposed bone area (**b**), and bony sequestration began at the posterior maxilla (stage 2) (arrow) (**c**). Exposed bone was surrounded by inflammatory granulation tissues and was easily sequestered from the host bone (**d**).

4

Antiresorptive Drug-related Osteonecrosis of the Jaw (ARONJ)—a Guide to Research   Kenneth E Fleisher, Risto Kontio, Sven Otto

recent classification system from the AAOMS in 2014 added the phrase "or fistulae that probes to bone" with exposed and necrotic bone in stages 1, 2, and 3 [14]. Therefore, some of the lesions that were previously graded stage 0 in the 2009 AAOMS position paper became classified as stage 2 or 3 according to the 2014 AAOMS position paper when there is evident necrotic bone lesion or sequestra, even in the absence of wide bone exposure (**Fig 1-2**). Therefore, it is clear that the recent AAOMS position paper confirmed the existence of the nonexposed variant of ONJ (stage 0) (**Table 1-2**).

The comparison of recently published reports from the 2014 AAOMS position paper [14] and the 2015 International Task Force on Osteonecrosis of the Jaw [27] is listed in **Table 1-3**. The major difference between these two is that the latter did not include the nonexposed type of lesion as ONJ.

Khan et al insisted that "exposed" bone should be included and did not regard necrotic bone with fistulous tract as ONJ [27]. A recent multicenter clinical study showed that up to a quarter of patients with ONJ associated with antiresorptive agents remained undiagnosed [31]. Therefore, the 2015 international task force has been criticized concerning issues of the potential risk of underestimation of ONJ [32]. However, the previously suggested staging system had not been confirmed to be correlated with the prognosis of the lesion. A higher grade does not definitively indicate the poor prognosis of the lesion [33]. A more refined classification is necessary to overcome the limitations in application to the clinical field.

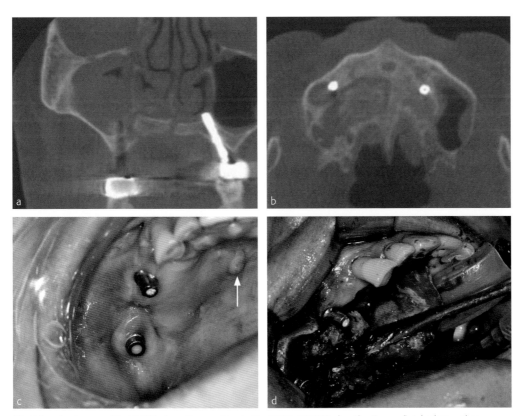

Fig 1-2a–d A case with ARONJ stage 3 according to the 2014 AAOMS classification: a fistula that probes to the bone in patients with infection extending beyond the region of the maxillary alveolar bone. A necrotic bone lesion was located under the nasal floor (**a, b**). Overlying palatal soft tissue was generally intact except the small fistula at mid palate (arrow) (**c**). The sequestra was composed of necrotic bone (**d**). This patient was administered ibandronate for 2.5 years to treat female osteoporosis.

	2007 AAOMS [10]	2009 AAOMS [13]	2014 AAOMS [14]
At risk	No apparent exposed/necrotic bone in patients that have been treated with either oral or IV BPs	No apparent necrotic bone in patients that have been treated with either oral or IV BPs	No apparent necrotic bone in patients that have been treated with either oral or IV BPs
Stage 0	-	No clinical evidence of necrotic bone, but nonspecific clinical findings and symptoms	No clinical evidence of necrotic bone, but nonspecific clinical findings and symptoms
Stage 1	Exposed/necrotic bone in patients that are asymptomatic and have no evidence of infection.	Exposed and necrotic bone in asymptomatic patients without evidence of infection	Exposed and necrotic bone, or fistulae that probes to bone, in patients that are asymptomatic and have no evidence of infection
Stage 2	Exposed/necrotic bone associated with infection as evidenced by pain and erythema in the region of the exposed bone with or without purulent drainage	Exposed and necrotic bone associated with infection as evidenced by pain and erythema in the region of exposed bone with or without purulent drainage	Exposed and necrotic bone, or fistulae that probes to bone, associated with infection as evidenced by pain and erythema in the region of the exposed bone with or without purulent drainage
Stage 3	Exposed/necrotic bone in patients with pain, infection, and one or more of the following: Pathologic fracture, extraoral fistula, or osteolysis extending to the inferior border of the mandible	Exposed and necrotic bone in patients with pain, infection, and one or more of the following: Exposed and necrotic bone extending beyond the region of alveolar bone, (ie, inferior border and ramus in the mandible, maxillary sinus, and zygoma in the maxilla) resulting in pathologic fracture, extraoral fistula, oral antral/oral nasal communication, or osteolysis extending to the inferior border of the mandible or sinus floor	Exposed and necrotic bone or fistulae that probes to bone in patients with pain, infection, and one or more of the following: Exposed and necrotic bone extending beyond the region of alveolar bone,(ie, inferior border and ramus in the mandible, maxillary sinus, and zygoma in the maxilla) resulting in pathologic fracture, extraoral fistula, oral antral/oral nasal communication, or osteolysis extending to the inferior border of the mandible or sinus floor

Table 1-2   Changes in staging proposed by the American Association of Oral and Maxillofacial Surgeons (AAOMS).

	2014 AAOMS position paper [14]	2015 International Task Force on Osteonecrosis of the Jaw [27]
At risk	No apparent necrotic bone in patients that have been treated with either oral or IV BP	-
Stage 0	No clinical evidence of necrotic bone, but nonspecific clinical findings and symptoms	-
Stage 1	Exposed and necrotic bone, or fistulae that probes to bone, in patients that are asymptomatic and have no evidence of infection	Asymptomatic, exposed bone on the mandible or maxilla, no evidence of significant adjacent or regional soft tissue inflammation or secondary infection
Stage 2	Exposed and necrotic bone, or fistulae that probes to bone, associated with infection as evidenced by pain and erythema in the region of the exposed bone with or without purulent drainage	Painful, exposed bone on mandible or maxilla, adjacent or regional soft tissue inflammation or secondary infection
Stage 3	Exposed and necrotic bone or fistulae that probes to bone in patients with pain, infection, and one or more of the following: exposed and necrotic bone extending beyond the region of alveolar bone,(ie, inferior border and ramus in the mandible, maxillary sinus, and zygoma in the maxilla) resulting in pathologic fracture, extraoral fistula, oral antral/oral nasal communication, or osteolysis extending to the inferior border of the mandible or sinus floor	Painful, exposed bone on mandible or maxilla, adjacent or regional soft tissue inflammation or secondary infection, extraoral fistula or oral antral fistula or radiographic evidence of osteolysis extending to the inferior border of the mandible or the floor of the maxillary sinus

Table 1-3   Comparison of the recent 2014 AAOMS position paper and the report from the 2015 International Task Force on Osteonecrosis of the Jaw.

5 Conclusion

Bone necrosis was first described by Professor James Russell from the University of Edinburg in 1794 to describe septic bone necrosis, but after the early 20th century, many scientists and clinicians recognized the existence of bone necrosis without septic condition. Until recently, osteonecrosis or aseptic necrosis was regarded as having the same meaning as ischemic or avascular necrosis. The definitions for ARONJ initially developed from the definition of osteoradionecrosis, which involved bone exposure for at least 2 months but as much as 6 months or more. From a 2006 Australian position paper to a 2009 AAOMS position paper, the definition of ARONJ was focused on ONJ after BP administration. From a 2011 American Dental Association definition, other antiresorptive or antiangiogenic agents (denosumab, bevacizumab, etc) were also included as causative agents of ONJ.

There have been a variety of terms and definitions for ARONJ suggested by various clinicians and academic societies. The variations of terminology reflect the status of understanding of ARONJ at a given time, which means that the whole field of ONJ is still developing. The current classification system of ARONJ supports the 2014 AAOMS definition of ONJ, which confirmed the existence of the nonexposed variant of ONJ. Established ARONJ without infection was regarded as stage 1, while stages 2 and 3 were categorized according to the severity of the infection and secondary complications.

6 References

1. **Nixon JE.** Avascular necrosis of bone: a review. *JR Soc Med.* 1983 Aug; 76(8):681–692.
2. **Marx RE.** Pamidronate (Aredia) and zoledronate (Zometa) induced avascular necrosis of the jaws: a growing epidemic. *J Oral Maxillofac Surg.* 2003 Sep; 61(9):1115–1117.
3. **Migliorati CA.** Bisphosphanates and oral cavity avascular bone necrosis. *J Clin Oncol.* 2003 Nov 15; 21(22):4253–4254.
4. **Harris M.** The conservative management of osteoradionecrosis of the mandible with ultrasound therapy. *Br J Oral Maxillofac Surg.* 1992 Oct; 30(5):313–318.
5. **Beumer J, Silverman S, Benak SB.** Hard and soft tissue necroses following radiation therapy for oral cancer. *J Prosthet Dent.* 1972 Jun; 27(6):640–644.
6. **Hutchinson IL.** Complications of radiotherapy in head and neck: an orofacial surgeon's view. In: Tobias JS, Thomas PR (eds). *Current Radiation Oncology.* London: Arnold; 1996:144–177.
7. **Marx RE.** Osteoradionecrosis: a new concept of its pathophysiology. *J Oral Maxillofac Surg.* 1983 May; 41(5):283–288.
8. **Sambrook P, Olver I, Goss A.** Bisphosphonates and osteonecrosis of the jaw. *Aust Fam Physician.* 2006 Oct; 35(10):801–803.
9. **Sambrook PN.** Consensus practice guidelines for bisphosphonate-associated osteonecrosis of the jaw. *Nat Clin Pract Rheumatol.* 2009 Jan; 5(1):6–7.
10. **American Association of Oral and Maxillofacial Surgeons.** Position paper on bisphosphonate-related osteonecrosis of the jaws. *J Oral Maxillofac Surg.* 2007 Mar; 65(3):369–376.
11. **Siddiqi A, Payne AG, Zafar S.** Bisphosphonate-induced osteonecrosis of the jaw: a medical enigma? *Oral Surg Oral Med Oral Pathol Oral Radiol Endod.* 2009 Sep; 108(3):e1–8.
12. **Khan AA, Sandor GK, Dore E, et al.** Canadian consensus practice guidelines for bisphosphonate associated osteonecrosis of the jaw. *J Rheumatol.* 2008 Jul; 35(7):1391–1397.
13. **Ruggiero SL, Dodson TB, Assael LA, et al.** American Association of Oral and Maxillofacial Surgeons position paper on bisphosphonate-related osteonecrosis of the jaw—2009 update. *Aust Endod J.* 2009 Dec; 35(3):119–130.
14. **Ruggiero SL, Dodson TB, Fantasia J, et al.** American Association of Oral and Maxillofacial Surgeons position paper on medication-related osteonecrosis of the jaw—2014 update. *J Oral Maxillofac Surg.* 2014 Oct; 72(10):1938–1956.
15. **Marx RE.** Bisphosphonate-induced osteonecrosis of the jaws: a challenge, a responsibility, and an opportunity. *Int J Periodontics Restorative Dent.* 2008 Feb; 28(1):5–6.
16. **Kelleher FC, McKenna M, Collins C, et al.** Bisphosphonate induced osteonecrosis of the jaws: unravelling uncertainty in disease causality. *Acta Oncol.* 2007; 46(5):702–704.
17. **Migliorati CA, Casiglia J, Epstein J, et al.** Managing the care of patients with bisphosphonate-associated osteonecrosis: an American Academy of Oral Medicine position paper. *J Am Dent Assoc.* 2005 Dec; 136(12):1658–1668.
18. **Khosla S, Burr D, Cauley J, et al.** Bisphosphonate-associated osteonecrosis of the jaw: report of a task force of the American Society for Bone and Mineral Research. *J Bone Miner Res.* 2007 Oct; 22(10):1479–1491.
19. **Wimalawansa SJ.** Bisphosphonate-associated osteomyelitis of the jaw: guidelines for practicing clinicians. *Endocr Pract.* 2008 Dec; 14(9):1150–1168.
20. **Yamazaki T, Takahashi K, Bessho K.** Recent Clinical Evidence in Bisphosphonate-related Osteomyelitis of the Jaw: Focus on Risk, Prevention and Treatment. *Rev Recent Clin Trials.* 2014; 9(1):37–52.
21. **Sihler KC, Chenoweth C, Zalewski C, et al.** Catheter-related vs. catheter-associated blood stream infections in the intensive care unit: incidence, microbiology, and implications. *Surg Infect (Larchmt).* 2010 Dec; 11(6):529–534.
22. **Hellstein JW, Adler RA, Edwards B, et al.** Managing the care of patients receiving antiresorptive therapy for prevention and treatment of osteoporosis: executive summary of recommendations from the American Dental Association Council on Scientific Affairs. *J Am Dent Assoc.* 2011 Nov; 142(11):1243–1251.
23. **Jones AC.** Recommendations questioned. *J Am Dent Assoc.* 2012 Jul; 143(7):732, 734; author reply 734.
24. **Diz P, Lopez-Cedrun JL, Arenaz J, et al.** Denosumab-related osteonecrosis of the jaw. *J Am Dent Assoc.* 2012 Sep; 143(9):981–984.
25. **Ristow O, Gerngross C, Schwaiger M, et al.** Effect of antiresorptive drugs on bony turnover in the jaw: denosumab compared with bisphosphonates. *Br J Oral Maxillofac Surg.* 2014 Apr; 52(4):308–313.

26. **Mignogna MD, Sadile G, Leuci S.** Drug-related osteonecrosis of the jaws: "Exposure, or not exposure: that is the question". *Oral Surg Oral Med Oral Pathol Oral Radiol.* 2012 May; 113(5):704–705.

27. **Khan AA, Morrison A, Hanley DA, et al.** Diagnosis and management of osteonecrosis of the jaw: a systematic review and international consensus. *J Bone Miner Res.* 2015 Jan; 30(1):3–23.

28. **Yoneda T, Hagino H, Sugimoto T, et al.** Bisphosphonate-related osteonecrosis of the jaw: position paper from the Allied Task Force Committee of Japanese Society for Bone and Mineral Research, Japan Osteoporosis Society, Japanese Society of Periodontology, Japanese Society for Oral and Maxillofacial Radiology, and Japanese Society of Oral and Maxillofacial Surgeons. *J Bone Miner Metab.* 2010 Jul; 28(4):365–383.

29. **Yarom N, Fedele S, Lazarovici TS, et al.** Is exposure of the jawbone mandatory for establishing the diagnosis of bisphosphonate-related osteonecrosis of the jaw? *J Oral Maxillofac Surg.* 2010 Mar; 68(3):705.

30. **Bedogni A, Fusco V, Agrillo A, et al.** Learning from experience. Proposal of a refined definition and staging system for bisphosphonate-related osteonecrosis of the jaw (BRONJ). *Oral Dis.* 2012 Sep; 18(6):621–623.

31. **Fedele S, Bedogni G, Scoletta M, et al.** Up to a quarter of patients with osteonecrosis of the jaw associated with antiresorptive agents remain undiagnosed. *Br J Oral Maxillofac Surg.* 2015 Jan; 53(1):13–17.

32. **Otto S, Marx RE, Troltzsch M, et al.** Comments on "diagnosis and management of osteonecrosis of the jaw: a systematic review and international consensus". *J Bone Miner Res.* 2015 Jun; 30(6):1113–1115.

33. **Otto S, Kwon T-G, Assaf AT.** Definition, clinical features and staging of medication-related osteonecrosis of the jaw. In: Otto S (ed). Medication-Related Osteonecrosis of the Jaws. Berlin Heidelberg: Springer; 2015:43–54.

2 Clinical features of antiresorptive drug-related osteonecrosis of the jaw

Morten Schiodt, Bente Brokstad Herlofson

1 Introductory questions

In this chapter, the following questions are raised and discussed:

- How do we take a medical history based on relevant factors?
- How do we diagnose and classify nonexposed osteonecrosis?
- How do we avoid misdiagnosing common dental infections like apical periodontal processes as nonexposed antiresorptive drug-related osteonecrosis of the jaw (ARONJ)?
- Is the development of ARONJ spontaneous or caused by a preceding trauma or dental procedure?
- What is the difference between ARONJ, osteomyelitis (OM), and osteoradionecrosis (ORN)?

2 Relevant anamnestic and clinical information

Well-prepared general and oral medical histories provide information pertinent to the diagnosis of ARONJ and aid in the identification of diseases, conditions, and comedications that increase the risk of this form of osteonecrosis of the jaw (ONJ). Because medication-related risk factors, local and anatomical factors, concomitant oral diseases, and demographic, systemic, genetic, and other medication factors have all been shown to contribute to the development of ONJ, it is vital to obtain and include these factors in the evaluation of these patients (**Figs 2-1, 2-2**) [1]. Unfortunately, many of these factors have been inconsistently reported as being key elements in the development of ARONJ. More research is therefore needed to validate the possible impact these factors have on the pathophysiology of this condition. However, it is a big challenge to acquire the information needed since most patients do not have a full overview of their own health history. Even medical records at hospitals can lack important data related to a patient's medical treatment [2, 3]. Without the correct medical information, providers can under-assess a patient's risk for the development of ARONJ. Much of this information comes from the patient's medical history, which can be practically divided into general medical history and oral medical history.

2.1   General medical history

Due to the challenge of obtaining a reliable general medical history, it is important for the evaluation and management of ARONJ patients to contact their general physician and/or other health personnel involved in their medical treatment, for any missing and corroborating information. Patients that develop ARONJ are predominately in the 35 to 95-year-old age group, with an average between 65 to 68 years [4–6]. In accordance with this, as most patients at risk for developing ONJ are older, validation of medical history information may be necessary. A patient-unique medication card would ease the medical history registration. Standard-ized health history forms (questionnaires) specifically developed for patients at risk may aid in gathering the medical history [3]. A clinical scale instrument that weighs the various risk factors to stratify risk for the development of ARONJ has been reported but needs further validation [7]. Potential issues in practical clinical work leading to under-diagnosing or late diagnosing include the fact that not all patients know the names of their antiresorptive medications, nor the relevant chemotherapy. Additionally, several co-morbid conditions and comedications have inconsistently been reported to be associated with ARONJ (**Fig 2-1**) [8–12].

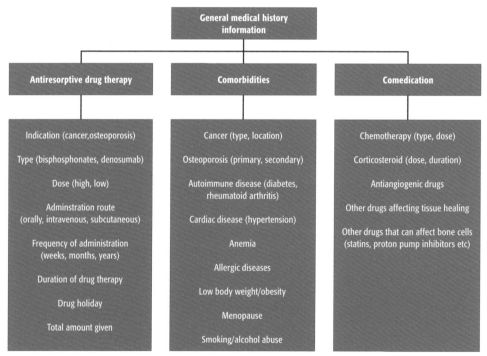

Fig 2-1   General medical information relevant in the health history evaluation of ARONJ patients or patients at risk for developing ARONJ.

2.2   Oral medical history

In addition to a thorough general medical history, a comprehensive review of the patient's oral and dental history is required. It has been shown that dentoalveolar surgery (such as tooth extraction), denture trauma, and periodontitis are related to the development of ONJ [1]. Oral events or oral diseases that could possibly be associated with the development of the ONJ condition should be addressed in the oral and dental history of the patient. There are important questions to address related to the oral events that occurred before ONJ was clinically established, such as what were the reasons for performing the dental procedure (extraction, endodontic therapy, periodontal treatment)? Could this have been associated with an early ONJ stage? But just as some information has been inconsistently reported as relevant in general medical history taking, so too has important data been inconsistently reported as relevant in developing oral health history evaluations (**Fig 2-2**).

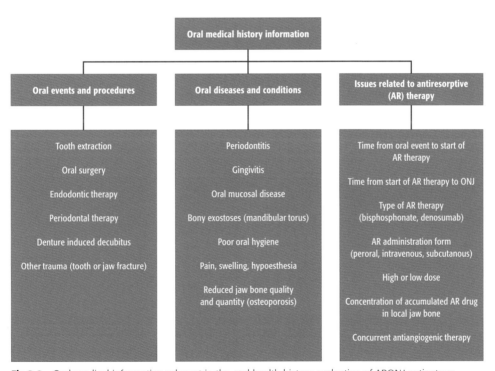

Fig 2-2   Oral medical information relevant in the oral health history evaluation of ARONJ patients or patients at risk for developing ARONJ.

3   Exposed or nonexposed variants of ARONJ

Antiresorptive drug-related osteonecrosis of the jaw is defined as the presence of exposed bone or bone that can be probed through an intraoral or extraoral fistula for more than 8 weeks in a patient on present or previous antiresorptive treatment, and who has no history of radiation to the jaws or obvious metastatic disease to the jaws (**Figs 2-3** to **2-7**) [1, 13–15]. This definition, initially introduced in 2006 [16], adjusted in 2009 [17], and 2014 [1], has won general acceptance.

However, it soon became clear that in addition to those ARONJ patients with exposed bone, there exists a condition termed "nonexposed" ARONJ (NE-ARONJ) [5, 18]. This patient group is characterized by the absence of clinically exposed bone but still has osteonecrosis (**Fig 2-5**) [13–15]. It was shown that the subgroups of exposed and nonexposed ARONJ did not differ from each other with regards to any relevant biologic parameter [5]. There are two subgroups of NE-ONJ, the first having a fistula through which the bone can be probed. This group, not recognized in the early 2006 and 2009 AAOMS consensus papers [16, 17] was subsequently recognized and incorporated into the 2014 AAOMS definition [1]. The official inclusion of this subgroup (with fistula) (**Fig 2-8**) [13–15] into the definition of "exposed bone" was a definite improvement in the clinical practical assessment and management of ARONJ patients.

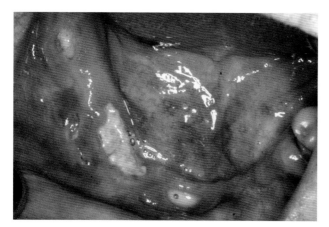

Fig 2-3   Stage 3 osteonecrosis, showing multiple areas of exposed bone in the mandible of an 82-year-old woman with breast cancer and metastases to the skeleton. She had been treated with zolendroic acid (zometa) for 30 months. Notice the pus formation anteriorly. The patient had impaired sensibility of the right mental nerve [13–15].

(Image with kind permission from the Danish, Norwegian, and Swedish Dental Journals).

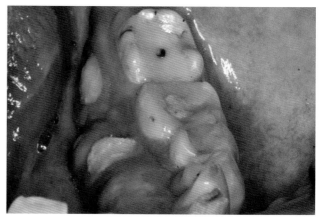

Fig 2-4   Osteonecrosis showing exposed bone corresponding to exostosis in the mandible (mandibular tori) in a 58-year-old woman with breast cancer and metastases treated with zolendroic acid (zometa) and ibandronate (bondronat) for 35 months [13–15].

(Image with kind permission from the Danish, Norwegian, and Swedish Dental Journals).

However, recognizing the subgroup of "true" NE-ONJ with no fistula and no exposed bone is still a diagnostic challenge (**Fig 2-9**) [5]. The AAOMS paper from 2009 [17] introduced an additional classification group called stage 0, defined as a patient on antiresorptive treatment and having nonspecific symptoms and/or changes or pathology and without clinical manifestations such as exposed bone. Research groups identified NE-ONJ and demonstrated that NE-ONJ may belong to the same disease entity as exposed ONJ [5, 18]. Recently, Fedele et al in a multicenter study demonstrated that up to one fourth of ONJ patients may actually have nonexposed ONJ [6]. It can then be argued that stage 0 includes both patients with "true" nonexposed ARONJ as well as patients that do not have developed ARONJ but are "at risk" [5]. **Table 2-1** outlines the various stages of ARONJ.

Several papers have suggested criteria for the diagnosis of nonexposed ARONJ, but at present there is no general consensus on any of these criteria, and they have not been validated in prospective scientific studies [5, 19]. So far, ARONJ is defined on medical history and clinical features [1]. The ultimate diagnosis of a nonexposed ARONJ may be the presence of necrotic bone on histology [5]. However, this is only feasible in retrospect when examining surgical specimens after resection. A bone biopsy for diagnosis before treatment is not considered practical as a routine procedure. However, the inclusion of imaging could be useful or even necessary in the diagnosis of those difficult cases of nonexposed ARONJ without fistulas [20–22].

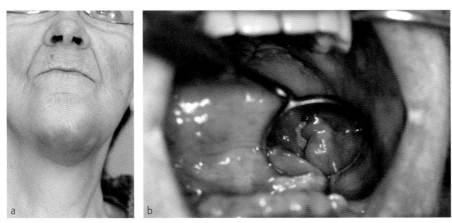

Fig 2-5a–b Osteonecrosis and submandibular abscess in a 72-year-old woman with multiple myeloma treated with pamidronate (aredia) for 114 months [13–15].
a Image showing the exposed bone of the left mandible.
b Intraoral view showing the submandibular abscess.

(Images with kind permission from the Danish, Norwegian, and Swedish Dental Journals).

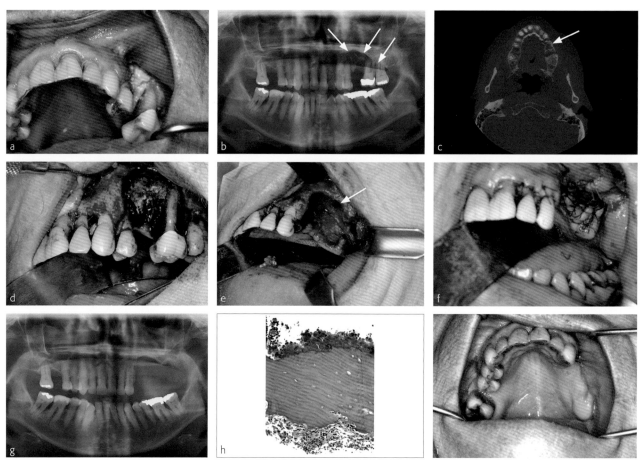

Fig 2-6a–i   The exposed bone of region 24–26 in a 62-year-old woman with osteoporosis, treated with alendronate for 84 months followed by denosumab (prolia) for 18 months, a total of 102 months on antiresorptive treatment. Tooth 25 had been removed 13 months earlier. Tooth 24 and 26 were mobile [13–15].
a   Exposed bone.
b   Section of a panoramic x-ray showing unhealed alveolus at tooth 25, and osteolysis in region 24–27 with central sequester (arrows).
c   Cone beam tomography showing sequester (arrow).
d   Intraoperative picture. Notice the green color of the dead bone.
e   Granulation tissue is removed revealing a small opening to the maxillary sinus (arrow). The palatal mucosa is exposed over a large area.
f   Primary closure. The patient had antibiotic treatment for 10 days postoperatively.
g   Postoperative control x-ray.
h   Histologic picture of removed specimen showing necrosis with empty osteocyte lacunae and bacteria on the surface.
i   Healing one month postoperatively. The patient was cured of the osteonecrosis and had function with a partial denture.

(Images with kind permission from the Danish, Norwegian, and Swedish Dental Journals, except Fig 2-6h, which is courtesy of Prof Jesper Reibel, Institute of Odontology, Copenhagen University).

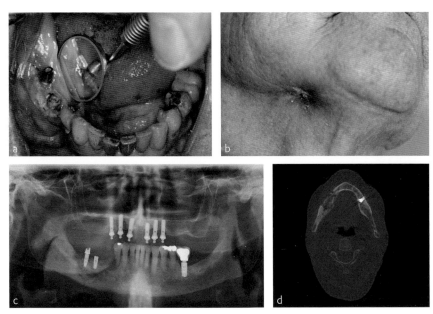

Fig 2-7a–d Osteonecrosis in the right mandible of a 67-year-old woman with osteoporosis treated with alendronate for 60 months [13–15].

a The patient had two dental implants inserted 2 years previously and had developed the present condition.

b Extraoral fistula with pus formation. Pain at level 7 on the visual analog scale (VAS) and decreased sensibility of right mentalis region. Osteonecrosis stage 3.

c Orthopan x-ray showing sequester formation in the right mandible.

d Cone beam tomography showing extensive osteonecrosis of the right mandible including fracture. The patient was treated with a continuity resection and reconstruction plate.

(Images with kind permission from the Danish, Norwegian, and Swedish Dental Journals).

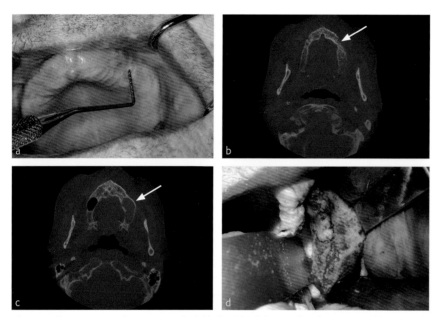

Fig 2-8a–d   Nonexposed osteonecrosis (with fistula) of the maxilla of a 69-year-old man with prostate cancer and metastases treated with denosumab (xgevar) for 19 months. The patient had pain in the left upper jaw [13–15].

a   The clinical view shows an apparently normal edentulous upper jaw. There is no exposed bone. On palpation, a small droplet of pus can be expelled through a nearly invisible fistula where the bone can be probed.

b   Cone beam scanning shows sequestrum at region 24–25 (arrow).

c   The infection also involved the left maxillary sinus (arrow).

d   Perioperative view showing osteonecrosis outlined on the bone surface. The process involved the maxillary sinus, which was cleaned and the wound closed with a flap of buccal fat pad, with mucosal closure on top. Uneventful healing was accomplished.

(Images with kind permission from the Danish, Norwegian, and Swedish Dental Journals).

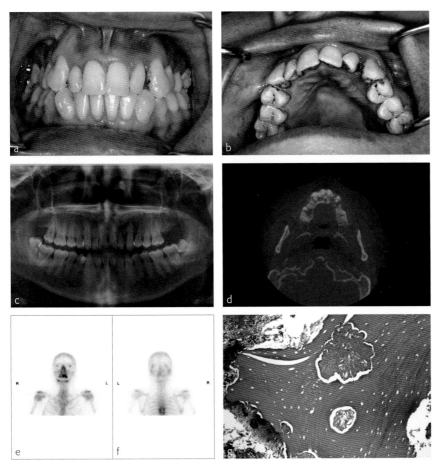

Fig 2-9a–g Nonexposed osteonecrosis (without fistula) of the jaws in a 41-year-old woman with breast cancer since 2003 and bone metastases since 2006, treated with zoledronic acid for 83 months [5].

a Note that there is no exposed bone or fistula. The maxillary left canine is rotated. The patient has pain. Classification: osteonecrosis stage 2, nonexposed osteonecrosis.

b Axial view showing a slight swelling of the alveolar process.

c Panoramic x-ray showing osteolysis and sequester formation in the alveolar process of the maxillary left canine region.

d Cone beam computed tomography of the patient showing sequester of the entire alveolar process to the palate.

e–f Scintigraphy showing signal from upper left anterior maxilla.

g Photomicrograph of sequester removed from the patient. Note the empty osteocyte lacunae and bacteria in marrow spaces.

(Images with kind permission from the Danish, Norwegian, and Swedish Dental Journals, except Fig 2-9g, which is courtesy of Prof Jesper Reibel, Institute of Odontology, Copenhagen University).

Patients at risk

No apparent necrotic bone in asymptomatic patients treated with intravenous or oral antiresorptive or antiangiogenic therapy.

Stage 0 (nonexposed bone variant)

Patients with no clinical evidence of necrotic bone but present with nonspecific symptoms or clinical and radiographic findings, such as the following:

Symptoms	**Clinical findings**	**Radiographic findings**
• Odontalgia not explained by an odontogenic cause • Dull aching bone pain in the body of the mandible, which may radiate to the temporomandibular joint region • Sinus pain, which may be associated with inflammation and thickening of the maxillary sinus wall • Altered neurosensory function.	• Loosening of teeth not explained by chronic periodontal disease • Periapical/periodontal fistula that is not associated with pulpal necrosis due to caries.	• Alveolar bone loss or resorption not attributable to chronic periodontal disease • Changes to trabecular pattern—dense woven bone and persistence of nonremodeled bone in extraction sockets • Regions of osteosclerosis involving the alveolar bone and/or the surrounding basilar bone • Thickening/obscuring of periodontal ligament (thickening of the lamina dura and decreased size of the periodontal ligament space).

These nonspecific findings, which characterize this nonexposed variant of ONJ, may occur in patients with a prior history of stage 1, 2, or 3 of the disease and who have healed and had no clinical evidence of exposed bone.

Stage 1

Exposed and necrotic bone, or fistulae that probe to bone, in patients that are asymptomatic and have no evidence of infection. These patients may also present with radiographic findings mentioned for stage 0 that are localized to the alveolar bone region.

Stage 2

Exposed and necrotic bone, or fistulae that probe to bone, with evidence of infection. These patients are typically symptomatic. These patients may also present with radiographic findings mentioned for stage 0 that are localized to the alveolar bone region.

Stage 3

Exposed and necrotic bone, or fistulae that probe to bone, with evidence of infection and one or more of the following:

• Exposed necrotic bone extending beyond the region of alveolar bone, ie, inferior border and ramus in the mandible, maxillary sinus, and zygoma in the maxilla
• Pathologic fracture
• Extraoral fistula
• Oral antral/oral nasal communication
• Osteolysis extending to the inferior border of the mandible or sinus floor.

Table 2-1   Stages of ARONJ [1].

4   Is the development of ARONJ spontaneous or caused by a preceding trauma or dental procedure?

Nearly all clinical series of ARONJ cases report that a trauma, most often tooth extraction, has preceded the onset of ARONJ. Additionally, denture trauma to the mucosa and oral surgery other than tooth extraction (eg, insertion of implants) can occur before the onset of ARONJ (**Fig 2-7**). The reported prevalence of trauma, notably tooth extraction, involves 50–70% of ARONJ patients [1, 23, 24]. In support of tooth extraction being an important cofactor or trigger factor for the onset of ARONJ is that mucosal healing after tooth extraction in patients on antiresorptive treatment is significantly slower than in patients not on antiresorptives [25]. Furthermore, experimental animal studies predictably produce ARONJ in animals on zoledronic acid after tooth extractions without soft tissue closure [26].

From the above figures, 30–50% of ARONJ cases are considered spontaneous; in most papers they account for around one-third. Many spontaneous ONJ lesions occur on the lingual aspect of the posterior mandible or on mandibular tori, which are covered by a thin oral mucosa and exhibit a different vascular system compared with other jaw areas (**Fig 2-4**). The anatomy of these areas facilitates vulnerability in the thin lingual oral mucosa. It might thus be speculated that a number of "spontaneous cases" are in fact also preceded by a traumatic event such as minor chewing trauma from hard food items exposed to the fragile mucosa, impressions trays, or intubation trauma in association with otherwise unrelated general anesthesia [23]. A number of papers have focused on the risk of ARONJ after planned (elective) tooth extractions. Most researchers recommend a tooth extraction combined with primary surgical mucosal closure of the alveolus on patients on high-dose antiresorptive treatment [27]. The prevalence of ARONJ after primary mucosal closure seems very low, around 2–5% [28–29].

5   Does the ARONJ process initiate as a bone or mucosal lesion or are both tissues involved?

The ambiguous question is: which tissue is affected first, the bone or the soft tissue, or are both initially involved (**Fig 2-10**)? Bisphosphonates are known to exert direct toxic effects to soft tissue cells, such as oral epithelial cells, and this can cause mucosal injury and exposed jaw bone [7, 30]. The consensus definition of medication-related ONJ has so far suggested that exposed bone is one of the key elements needed to achieve an ONJ diagnosis [1]. This definition has recently been challenged [5, 18]. Nonexposed variants of ONJ have been reported, which may indicate that the ONJ condition in some cases can start in bone tissue and that the soft tissue is affected afterwards (**Fig 2-9**). Soft tissue healing is shown to be delayed after surgical procedures such as tooth extraction in patients receiving bisphosphonates, however, this may not always result in jawbone exposure and ONJ [25, 31].

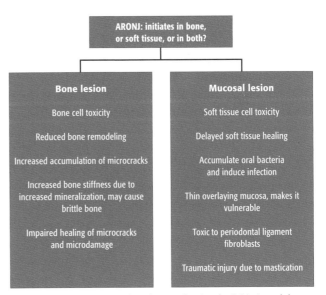

Fig 2-10   Factors to consider when evaluating the initiation of the ARONJ process; in bone, or soft tissue, or in both tissues at the same time.

6   Comparison between osteoradionecrosis, osteomyelitis, and ARONJ.

Exposed and/or necrotic jaw bone has been associated with several conditions, including zoster infection of the mandible and maxilla, yet some cases have occurred without a trigger course [32]. In one particular study, 60 extreme cases of osteonecrosis and osteomyelitis were reported from West Africa [33]. However, the three most common types of osteonecrosis of the jaw are osteoradionecrosis (ORN) related to irradiation, suppurative osteomyelitis (OM) related to infection, and osteonecrosis related to medication such as antiresorptive and antiangiogenic drugs (ARONJ). Conditions and diseases, treatments, and medications can alter the vascularity of bone and soft tissue, increasing the risk for ONJ development as seen with radiotherapy and the use of antiresorptive and antiangiogenic drugs in cancer and osteoporosis therapy. Clinically, the three entities of ORN, OM, and ARONJ can present with similar clinical features such as exposed bone, infection, fistulation, abscess formation, sequestration, and pathologic fracture [34–36]. Despite any clinical similarity, histopathological differences have been reported [34, 37] (**Table 2-2**).

6.1   Osteoradionecrosis

Osteoradionecrosis is related to radiation and defined as exposed bone that fails to heal over a period of 3 months or longer, worsens slowly, and does not heal spontaneously [38]. A variant of ORN, a nonexposed type without any breach of the oral mucosa or cervicofacial skin, has also been identified [38].

6.2   Osteomyelitis

Osteomyelitis is known as an inflammatory condition of the bone that begins as an infection of the medullary bone cavity, involving the Haversian systems, and extends to the periosteum of the affected area. Osteomyelitis is classified as either acute or chronic based on time. Chronic OM may show a suppuration course with abscess formation, and exposed bone can occur [39–41].

6.3   Antiresorptive drug-related osteonecrosis of the jaw

Antiresorptive drug-related osteonecrosis of the jaw is defined as the presence of exposed bone or bone that can be probed through an intraoral or extraoral fistula for more than 8 weeks in a patient on present or previous antiresorptive treatment or angiogenic inhibitors and who has no history of radiation to the jaws or obvious metastatic disease to the jaw [1]. **Table 2-2** provides a comparison of the various clinical features of ORN, OM, and ARONJ.

ORN related to radiation	OM related to infection	ARONJ related to medication
Tissue becomes hypovascular, hypocellular, hypoxic	Bone becomes infected via local infected tissue or via the bloodstream	Bisphosphonates accumulate in jaw bone
Bone marrow replaced with fibrotic tissue	Increased number of inflammatory cells	Toxic effect to bone and soft tissue cells
Limited inflammatory cell infiltration	Bone marrow inflammation and vessel thrombosis	Suppression of local bone blood supply
Nonviable periosteum, no evidence of reactive bone formation	May show periosteal bone formation	May show viable periosteum and reactive bone formation
Almost entirely in the mandible	Most often in the mandible	2/3 of cases in the mandible

Table 2-2   Features of osteoradionecrosis (ORN), osteomyelitis (OM), and antiresorptive drug-related osteonecrosis of the jaw (ARONJ) with similar clinical manifestations.

7   Conclusion

Well documented patient medical histories that include both general medical and oral and dental history are important to ensure medical caregivers can better assess a patient's risk for developing ARONJ. However, practitioners should be aware that both general and oral medical information has been inconsistently reported to be relevant in the evaluation of patients at risk for ARONJ. What has been shown is that ARONJ cases often undergo tooth extraction or experience an infection preceding the onset of ARONJ. A comparison of features related to ORN, OM, and ARONJ that have similar clinical manifestations has been provided.

8   References

1. **Ruggiero SL, Dodson TB, Fantasia J, et al.** American Association of Oral and Maxillofacial Surgeons position paper on medication-related osteonecrosis of the jaw—2014 update. *J Oral Maxillofac Surg.* 2014 Oct; 72(10):1938–1956.
2. **Landesberg R, Taxel P.** Osteonecrosis of the jaw and rheumatoid arthritis. Is it the disease or the drugs? *J Rheumatol.* 2013 Jun; 40(6):749–751.
3. **Schiodt M, Wexell CL, Herlofson BB, et al.** Existing data sources for clinical epidemiology: Scandinavian Cohort for osteonecrosis of the jaw—work in progress and challenges. *Clin Epidemiol.* 2015 Jan; 7:107–116.
4. **Kuhl S, Walter C, Acham S, et al.** Bisphosphonate-related osteonecrosis of the jaws—a review. *Oral Oncol.* 2012 Oct; 48(10):938–947.
5. **Schiodt M, Reibel J, Oturai P, et al.** Comparison of nonexposed and exposed bisphosphonate-induced osteonecrosis of the jaws: a retrospective analysis from the Copenhagen cohort and a proposal for an updated classification system. *Oral Surg Oral Med Oral Pathol Oral Radiol.* 2014 Feb; 117(2):204–213.
6. **Fedele S, Bedogni G, Scoletta M, et al.** Up to a quarter of patients with osteonecrosis of the jaw associated with antiresorptive agents remain undiagnosed. *Br J Oral Maxillofac Surg.* 2015 Jan; 53(1):13–17.
7. **Landesberg R, Woo V, Cremers S, et al.** Potential pathophysiological mechanisms in osteonecrosis of the jaw. *Ann NY Acad Sci.* 2011 Feb; 1218:62–79.
8. **Marx RE, Sawatari Y, Fortin M, et al.** Bisphosphonate-induced exposed bone (osteonecrosis/osteopetrosis) of the jaws: risk factors, recognition, prevention, and treatment. *J Oral Maxillofac Surg.* 2005 Nov; 63(11):1567–1575.
9. **Sawatari Y, Marx RE.** Bisphosphonates and bisphosphonate induced osteonecrosis. *Oral Maxillofac Surg Clin North Am.* 2007 Nov; 19(4):487–498.
10. **Thumbigere-Math V, Tu L, Huckabay S, et al.** A retrospective study evaluating frequency and risk factors of osteonecrosis of the jaw in 576 cancer patients receiving intravenous bisphosphonates. *Am J Clin Oncol.* 2012 Aug; 35(4):386–392.
11. **Wessel JH, Dodson TB, Zavras AI.** Zoledronate, smoking, and obesity are strong risk factors for osteonecrosis of the jaw: a case-control study. *J Oral Maxillofac Surg.* 2008 Apr; 66(4):625–631.

12. **Saad F, Brown JE, Van Poznak C, et al.** Incidence, risk factors, and outcomes of osteonecrosis of the jaw: integrated analysis from three blinded active-controlled phase III trials in cancer patients with bone metastases. *Ann Oncol.* 2012 May; 23(5):1341–1347.
13. **Schiodt M, Wexell CL, Herlofson BB, et al.** Medicinrelateret osteonekrose i kæberne—oversigt og retningslinjer. *Tandlaegebladet [Danish Dental Journal].* 2015; 119:918–930. Danish.
14. **Herlofson BB, Wexell CL, Norholt SE et al.** Medikamentrelatert osteonekrose i kjevene. Del 1:oversikt og retningslinjer. *Nor Tannlegeforen Tid [Norwegian Dental Journal].* 2015; 125:880–890. Norwegian.
15. **Wexell CL, Herlofson BB, Norholt SE et al.** Läkemedelsrelaterad osteonekros i käkarna, del 1:Översikt och riktlinjer. *Tandläkartidningen [Swedish Dental Journal].* 2015; 107(12):112–123. Swedish.
16 **Ruggiero SL, Fantasia J, Carlson E.** Bisphosphonate-related osteonecrosis of the jaw: background and guidelines for diagnosis, staging and management. *Oral Surg Oral Med Oral Pathol Oral Radiol.* 2006 Oct; 102(4):433–441.
17. **Ruggiero SL, Dodson TB, Assael LA, et al.** American Association of Oral and Maxillofacial Surgeons position paper on bisphosphonate-related osteonecrosis of the jaws—2009 update. *J Oral Maxillofac Surg.* 2009 May; 67(5 Suppl):S2–12.
18. **Fedele S, Porter SR, D'Aiuto F, et al.** Nonexposed variant of bisphosphonate-associated osteonecrosis of the jaw: a case series. *Am J Med.* 2010 Nov; 123(11):1060–1064.
19 **Bagan J, Scully C, Sabater V, et al.** Osteonecrosis of the jaws in patients treated with intravenous bisphosphonates (BRONJ): A concise update. *Oral Oncol.* 2009 July; 45:551–554.
20. **Bedogni A, Fedele S, Bedogni G, et al.** Staging of osteonecrosis of the jaw requires computed tomography for accurate definition of the extent of bony disease. *Br J Oral Maxillofac Surg.* 2014 Sep; 52(7):603–608.
21. **Franco S, Miccoli S, Limongelli L, et al.** New dimensional staging of bisphosphonate-related osteonecrosis of the jaw allowing a guided surgical treatment protocol: long-term follow-up of 266 lesions in neoplastic and osteoporotic patients from the university of bari. *Int J Dent.* 2014; doi:10.1155/2014/935657. Epub 6/5/2014.

22. **Miyashita H, Shiba H, Kawana H, et al.** Clinical utility of three-dimensional SPECT/CT imaging as a guide for the resection of medication-related osteonecrosis of the jaw. *Int J Oral Maxillofac Surg.* 2015 Sep; 44(9):1106–1109.

23. **Yazdi PM, Schiodt M.** Dentoalveolar trauma and minor trauma as precipitating factors for medication-related osteonecrosis of the jaw (ONJ): a retrospective study of 149 consecutive patients from the Copenhagen ONJ Cohort. *Oral Surg Oral Med Oral Pathol Oral Radiol.* 2015 Apr; 119(4):416–422.

24. **Campisi G, Fedele S, Fusco V, et al.** Epidemiology, clinical manifestations, risk reduction and treatment strategies of jaw osteonecrosis in cancer patients exposed to antiresorptive agents. *Future Oncol.* 2014 Feb; 10(2):257–275.

25. **Migliorati C, Saunders D, Conlou MS, et al.** Assessing the association between bisphosphonate exposure and delayed mucosal healing after tooth extraction. *JADA.* 2013 Apr; 144(4):406–414.

26. **Sharma D, Hamlet S, Petcu E, et al.** Animal models for bisphosphonate-related osteonecrosis of the jaws—an appraisal. *Oral Dis.* 2013 Nov; 19(8):747–754.

27. **Saia G, Blandamura S, Bettini G, et al.** Occurrence of bisphosphonate-related osteonecrosis of the jaw after surgical tooth extraction. *J Oral Maxillofac Surg.* 2010 Apr; 68(4):797–804.

28. **Ferlito S, Puzzo S, Liardo C.** Preventive protocol for tooth extractions in patients treated with zoledronate: a case series. *J Oral Maxillofac Surg.* 2011 Jun; 69(6):e1–4.

29. **Otto S, Troltzsch M, Jambrovic V, et al.** Tooth extraction in patients receiving oral or intravenous bisphosphonate administration: A trigger for BRONJ development? *J Craniomaxillofac Surg.* 2015 Jul; 43(6):847–854.

30. **Landesberg R, Cozin M, Cremers S, et al.** Inhibition of oral mucosal cell wound healing by bisphosphonates. *J Oral Maxillofac Surg.* 2008 May; 66(5):839–847.

31. **Fehm T, Beck V, Banys M, et al.** Bisphosphonate-induced osteonecrosis of the jaw (ONJ): Incidence and risk factors in patients with breast cancer and gynecological malignancies. *Gynecol Oncol.* 2009 Mar; 112(3):605–609.

32. **Schiodt M.** Herpes zoster related osteonecrosis of the jaws. Consequences for implant treatment? Presented at: International Association for Oral and Maxillofacial Surgery Biannual Congress. Oct 30–Nov 4, 2011; Santiago, Chile.

33. **Khullar SM, Tvedt D, Chapman K, et al.** Sixty cases of extreme osteonecrosis and osteomyelitis of the mandible and maxilla in a West African population. *Int J Oral Maxillofac Surg.* 2012 Aug; 41:978–985.

34. **Marx RE, Tursun R.** Suppurative osteomyelitis, bisphosphonate induced osteonecrosis, osteoradionecrosis: a blinded histopathologic comparison and its implications for the mechanism of each disease. *Int J Oral Maxillofac Surg.* 2012 Mar; 41(3):283–289.

35. **Prasad KC, Prasad SC, Mouli N, et al.** Osteomyelitis in the head and neck. *Acta Otolaryngol.* 2007 Feb; 127(2):194–205.

36. **Hoefert S, Schmitz I, Weichert F, et al.** Macrophages and bisphosphonate-related osteonecrosis of the jaw (BRONJ): evidence of local immunosuppression of macrophages in contrast to other infectious jaw diseases. *Clin Oral Investig.* 2015 Mar; 19(2):497–508.

37. **Mitsimponas KT, Moebius P, Amann K, et al.** Osteo-radio-necrosis (ORN) and bisphosphonate-related osteonecrosis of the jaws (BRONJ): the histopathological differences under the clinical similarities. *Int J Clin Exp Pathol.* 2014 Jan; 7(2):496–508.

38. **Store G, Boysen M.** Mandibular osteoradionecrosis: clinical behaviour and diagnostic aspects. *Clin Otolaryngol Allied Sci.* 2000 Oct; 25(5):378–384.

39. **Suei Y, Taguchi A, Tanimoto K.** Diagnosis and classification of mandibular osteomyelitis. *Oral Surg Oral Med Oral Pathol Oral Radiol.* 2005 Aug; 100(2):207–214.

40. **Baur DA, Altay MA, Flores-Hidalgo A, et al.** Chronic osteomyelitis of the mandible: diagnosis and management—an institution's experience over 7 years. *J Oral Maxillofac Surg.* 2015 Apr; 73(4):655–665.

41. **Di Fiore PM, Cerrud CC, Buckley IA, et al.** Osteomyelitis of the mandible in an adolescent. *J Dent Child.* 2015 May; 82(2):102–107.

3 Imaging modalities for antiresorptive drug-related osteonecrosis of the jaw

Kenneth E Fleisher, King Chong Chan, Niloufar Amintavakoli

1 Introductory questions

In this chapter, the following questions are raised and discussed:
- Which imaging modalities are used for the diagnosis of antiresorptive drug-related osteonecrosis of the jaw (ARONJ)?
- What are the advantages and disadvantages of each imaging modality?
- What are the radiographic findings for ARONJ?
- What is meant by metabolic changes for ARONJ lesions?

2 Conventional imaging

Although the radiographic changes for ARONJ are nonspecific, they provide valuable information on the course, magnitude, and progression of ARONJ [1, 2]. While panorex radiography is considered the standard imaging for oral and maxillofacial surgery, it tends to underestimate the extent of ARONJ lesions compared with computed tomography (CT) imaging [3, 4]. The advantages of cone beam computed tomography (CBCT) compared with multiple detector computed tomography (MDCT) include higher spatial resolution, better image quality, lower radiation dose, and lower cost [5]. Together, a number of common findings present themselves when using radiography, CBCT, and MDCT [1, 3, 4, 6–9] (**Figs 3-1** to **3-3**), which include the following:
- Osteolysis
- Osteosclerosis
- Bone sequestra (bone-within-bone appearance)
- Cortical disruption
- Periosteal reaction
- Delayed or absent bone remodeling at extraction sites
- Thickened lamina dura
- Pathologic fracture.

3 Magnetic resonance imaging

While magnetic resonance imaging (MRI) is free of ionizing radiation, allows for the evaluation of bone marrow changes, and can identify osteomyelitis in the acute stages before bony changes are visualized by plain radiography [1], its limitations include an inability to visualize the destruction of cortical bone [10, 11], an inability to distinguish edema from infection [12], and the inability to identify ARONJ lesions [13]. Magnetic resonance imaging findings are provided through the following [1, 2, 7, 14]:
- T1-weighted imaging: low signal intensity
- T2-weighted imaging: increased signal intensity in early disease; variable signal intensity in later disease. Signals can be intermediate or slightly increased in early disease when features of acute inflammation (edema, hypervascularity) dominate. Signals may be low in late disease when features of chronic inflammation (fibrosis, hypovascularity) dominate
- Low intensity in the sequestrum in both T1- and T2-weighted images. Low T1- and T2-weighted signal in exposed bone; low T1 signal in unexposed affected bone [2]
- Gadolinium-enhanced imaging: rim enhancement in areas adjacent to necrotic bone [1, 2].

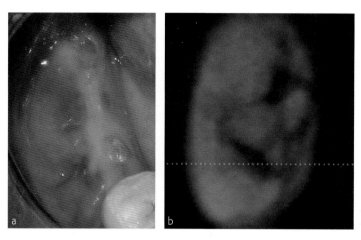

Fig 3-1a–b   A clinical image showing ARONJ with fistula of the right mandible (**a**) and the CBCT indicating sequestrum of the right mandible and osteosclerosis (**b**).

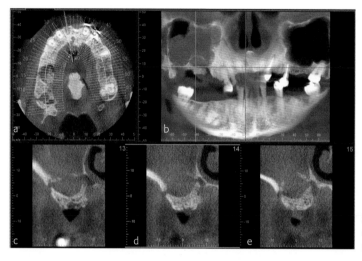

Fig 3-2a–e   A CBCT of a patient's maxilla with axial, coronal, and panoramic views demonstrating sequestration of the right alveolus sinus floor and fluid in the maxillary sinus.

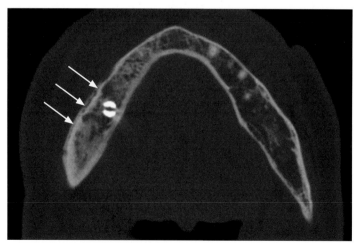

Fig 3-3   An axial CBCT view of a mandible illustrating subperiosteal bone reaction on the lateral cortex and diffuse osteosclerosis of the right mandible (arrows).

4 Nuclear imaging

Conventional imaging with periapical or panoramic radiographs, CT, and/or MRI exhibit little or no change in bony architecture in the early stages of ARONJ, only visualize lesions after structural changes have taken place, often underestimate the amount of necrotic bone, and may not represent metabolic changes due to increased cellular metabolic activity during inflammation [15–21]. Additional nuclear imaging may therefore be beneficial.

4.1 Nuclear bone scintigraphy

Nuclear bone scintigraphy with technetium and single photon emission computed tomography (SPECT) is another imaging modality that can identify early, subclinical, and stage 0 ARONJ lesions [10, 18]. Tracer uptake is dependent on increased blood flow (ie, inflammation) and new bone formation (ie, increased osteoblastic activity and mineral turnover) [22]. Nuclear imaging quality can be enhanced using fused SPECT [23] and facilitates the differentiation between increased uptake of reactive bone and decreased uptake of bone sequestra [14].

4.2 Fluorodeoxyglucose positron emission tomography

Fluorodeoxyglucose positron emission tomography with computed tomography (FDG PET-CT) has become the standard imaging procedure in the management of metastatic breast cancer, and is used to detect distant metastasis and recurrence, to screen for extra-axillary drainage sites, and to assess the response to neoadjuvant chemotherapy [24]. The use of FDG PET-CT is widely accepted as a sensitive imaging technique in the diagnosis, staging, and management of multiple myeloma [25, 26]. Fluorodeoxyglucose used for PET scans accumulates not only in malignant tissues but at sites of increased metabolic activity due to infection and inflammation [27, 28]. Combining FDG PET and CT scans merges anatomical and metabolic findings [29]. The presence of inflammatory dental disease appears to be a risk factor for developing ARONJ in more than 50% of cases, suggesting that tooth extraction might be incidental rather than the precipitant [30-32]. Studies are needed to compare nuclear imaging techniques (**Fig 3-4**).

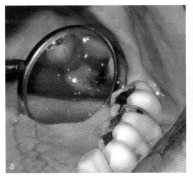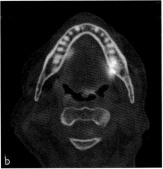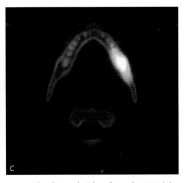

Fig 3-4a–c Clinical image showing ARONJ of the left mandible with exposed bone on the lingual side of tooth #18 (**a**). Nuclear imaging using FDG PET-CT with localized FDG uptake (**b**). A technetium bone scan indicating diffuse osteoblast changes in the left mandible (**c**).

A retrospective study by Fleisher et al of 25 clinically identified medication-related ONJ lesions were analyzed using radiography and FDG PET-CT [33]. Differences were found in how radiography and FDG PET-CT detect local and diffuse changes associated with ARONJ. Radiography showed local changes in 17 patients (68%), diffuse changes in three patients (12%), and no changes in five patients (20%). However, FDG PET-CT imaging showed local changes in 25 patients (100%) and diffuse changes in eight patients (32%). The results of this study illustrates that FDG PET-CT detects local and diffuse metabolic changes that may not be represented by plain radiography for patients with ARONJ related to antiresorptive therapy.

This information may facilitate surgical management decisions and improve outcomes [34]. Use of 18F-sodium fluoride positron emission tomography with computed tomography (NaF PET-CT) can also detect subtle foci of increased bone remodeling not visible on anatomical imaging [1, 13, 19].

Stage 0 ARONJ is characterized by an absence of clinically exposed bone in patients presenting with nonspecific symptoms or clinical and radiographic findings. Panorex, CBCT, and CT imaging may be significant for sequestra, osteosclerosis, osteolysis, cortical bone disruption, prominence of the inferior alveolar nerve canal, unremodeled bone at an extraction site, and widening of periodontal ligament space [9, 35, 36] (**Fig 3-5**). Bone scintigraphy can help to identify subclinical ARONJ that subsequently progresses to frank bone exposure [18]. Up to 50% of patients with clinically diagnosed stage 0 could progress to frank bone exposure [37].

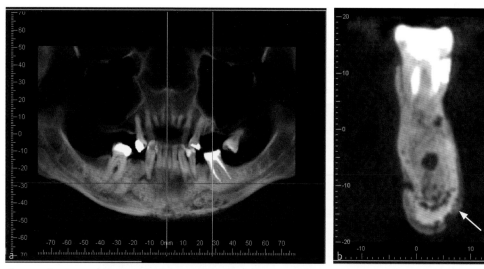

Fig 3-5a–b   Stage 0 ARONJ of the left mandible. The CBCT shows diffuse osteosclerosis and osteolysis of the mandible (**a**). A coronal section through the mandibular left first molar shows osteolytic changes and subperiosteal bone formation along the lateral and medial cortices (arrow) (**b**).

5 Conclusion

Radiographic imaging is commonly used for the screening of patients at risk or diagnosed with ARONJ. Use of CT or CBCT imaging modalities is preferred for surgical treatment planning to identify subclinical structural bone changes and extension of ARONJ lesions. Nuclear imaging with FDG PET-CT can further contribute towards understanding subclinical bone changes to improve surgical outcomes. Further research is needed to determine if FDG PET-CT imaging can detect risk and the early stages of ARONJ.

6 References

1. **Arce K, Assael LA, Weissman JL, et al.** Imaging findings in bisphosphonate-related osteonecrosis of jaws. *J Oral Maxillofac Surg.* 2009 May; 67(5 Suppl):S75–84.
2. **Bisdas S, Chambron Pinho N, Smolarz A, et al.** Biphosphonate-induced osteonecrosis of the jaws: CT and MRI spectrum of findings in 32 patients. *Clin Radiol.* 2008 Jan; 63(1):71–77.
3. **Bedogni A, Blandamura S, Lokmic Z, et al.** Bisphosphonate-associated jawbone osteonecrosis: a correlation between imaging techniques and histopathology. *Oral Surg Oral Med Oral Pathol Oral Radiol Endod.* 2008 Mar; 105(3):358–364.
4. **Bianchi SD, Scoletta M, Cassione FB, et al.** Computerized tomographic findings in bisphosphonate-associated osteonecrosis of the jaw in patients with cancer. *Oral Surg Oral Med Oral Pathol Oral Radiol Endod.* 2007 Aug; 104(2):249–258.
5. **Khosla S, Burr D, Cauley J, et al.** Bisphosphonate-associated osteonecrosis of the jaw: report of a task force of the American Society for Bone and Mineral Research. *J Bone Miner Res.* 2007 Oct; 22(10):1479–1491.
6. **Fatterpekar GM, Emmrich JV, Eloy JA, et al.** Bone-within-bone appearance: a red flag for biphosphonate-associated osteonecrosis of the jaw. *J Comput Assist Tomogr.* 2011 Sep-Oct; 35(5):553–556.
7. **Haworth AE, Webb J.** Skeletal complications of bisphosphonate use: what the radiologist should know. *Br J Radiol.* 2012 Oct; 85(1018):1333–1342.
8. **Wilde F, Heufelder M, Lorenz K, et al.** Prevalence of cone beam computed tomography imaging findings according to the clinical stage of bisphosphonate-related osteonecrosis of the jaw. *Oral Surg Oral Med Oral Pathol Oral Radiol.* 2012 Dec; 114(6):804–811.
9. **Hutchinson M, O'Ryan F, Chavez V, et al.** Radiographic findings in bisphosphonate-treated patients with stage 0 disease in the absence of bone exposure. *J Oral Maxillofac Surg.* 2010 Sep; 68(9):2232–2240.
10. **Chiandussi S, Biasotto M, Dore F, et al.** Clinical and diagnostic imaging of bisphosphonate-associated osteonecrosis of the jaws. *Dentomaxillofac Radiol.* 2006 Jul; 35(4):236–243.
11. **Dore F, Filippi L, Biasotto M, et al.** Bone scintigraphy and SPECT/CT of bisphosphonate-induced osteonecrosis of the jaw. *J Nucl Med.* 2009 Jan; 50(1):30–35.
12. **Coviello V, Stevens MR.** Contemporary concepts in the treatment of chronic osteomyelitis. *Oral Maxillofac Surg Clin North Am.* 2007 Nov; 19(4):523–534, vi.
13. **Raje N, Woo SB, Hande K, et al.** Clinical, radiographic, and biochemical characterization of multiple myeloma patients with osteonecrosis of the jaw. *Clin Cancer Res.* 2008 Apr 15; 14(8):2387–2395.
14. **Morag Y, Morag-Hezroni M, Jamadar DA, et al.** Bisphosphonate-related osteonecrosis of the jaw: a pictorial review. *Radiographics.* 2009 Nov; 29(7):1971–1984.
15. **Fantasia JE.** Bisphosphonates—what the dentist needs to know: practical considerations. *J Oral Maxillofac Surg.* 2009 May; 67(5 Suppl):S53–60.
16. **Ruggiero S, Gralow J, Marx RE, et al.** Practical guidelines for the prevention, diagnosis, and treatment of osteonecrosis of the jaw in patients with cancer. *J Oncol Pract.* 2006 Jan; 2(1):7–14.
17. **Pazianas M, Russell RG, Fogelman I.** Osteonecrosis of the jaw: more heat than light. *J Nucl Med.* 2009 Jan; 50(1):6–7.
18. **O'Ryan FS, Khoury S, Liao W, et al.** Intravenous bisphosphonate-related osteonecrosis of the jaw: bone scintigraphy as an early indicator. *J Oral Maxillofac Surg.* 2009 Jul; 67(7):1363–1372.
19. **Guggenberger R, Fischer DR, Metzler P, et al.** Bisphosphonate-induced osteonecrosis of the jaw: comparison of disease extent on contrast-enhanced MR imaging, [18F] fluoride PET/CT, and conebeam CT imaging. *AJNR Am J Neuroradiol.* 2013 Jun-Jul; 34(6):1242–1247.
20. **Engroff SL, Kim DD.** Treating bisphosphonate osteonecrosis of the jaws: is there a role for resection and vascularized reconstruction? *J Oral Maxillofac Surg.* 2007 Nov; 65(11):2374–2385.
21. **Basu S, Chryssikos T, Moghadam-Kia S, et al.** Positron emission tomography as a diagnostic tool in infection: present role and future possibilities. *Semin Nucl Med.* 2009 Jan; 39(1):36–51.
22. **Palestro CJ, Love C.** Radionuclide imaging of musculoskeletal infection: conventional agents. *Semin Musculoskelet Radiol.* 2007 Dec; 11(4):335–352.
23. **Miyashita H, Shiba H, Kawana H, et al.** Clinical utility of three-dimensional SPECT/CT imaging as a guide for the resection of medication-related osteonecrosis of the jaw. *Int J Oral Maxillofac Surg.* 2015 Sep; 44(9):1106–1109.
24. **Groheux D, Giacchetti S, Rubello D, et al.** The evolving role of PET/CT in breast cancer. *Nucl Med Commun.* 2010 Apr; 31(4):271–273.

25. **Agarwal A, Chirindel A, Shah BA, et al.** Evolving role of FDG PET/CT in multiple myeloma imaging and management. *AJR Am J Roentgenol.* 2013 Apr; 200(4):884–890.

26. **Nanni C, Zamagni E, Celli M, et al.** The value of 18F-FDG PET-CT after autologous stem cell transplantation (ASCT) in patients affected by multiple myeloma (MM): experience with 77 patients. *Clin Nucl Med.* 2013 Feb; 38(2):e74–79.

27. **Meller J, Sahlmann CO, Liersch T, et al.** Nonprosthesis orthopedic applications of (18)F fluoro-2-deoxy-D-glucose PET in the detection of osteomyelitis. *Radiol Clin North Am.* 2007 Jul; 45(4):719–733, vii-viii.

28. **Israel O, Keidar Z.** PET/CT imaging in infectious conditions. *Ann NY Acad Sci.* 2011 Jun; 1228:150–166.

29. **Kalles V, Zografos GC, Provatopoulou X, et al.** The current status of positron emission mammography in breast cancer diagnosis. *Breast Cancer.* 2013 Apr; 20(2):123–130.

30. **Tsao C, Darby I, Ebeling PR, et al.** Oral health risk factors for bisphosphonate-associated jaw osteonecrosis. *J Oral Maxillofac Surg.* 2013 Aug; 71(8):1360–1366.

31. **Saad F, Brown JE, Van Poznak C, et al.** Incidence, risk factors, and outcomes of osteonecrosis of the jaw: integrated analysis from three blinded active-controlled phase III trials in cancer patients with bone metastases. *Ann Oncol.* 2012 May; 23(5):1341–1347.

32. **Adornato MC, Morcos I, Rozanski J.** The treatment of bisphosphonate-associated osteonecrosis of the jaws with bone resection and autologous platelet-derived growth factors. *J Am Dent Assoc.* 2007 Jul; 138(7):971–977.

33. **Fleisher KE, Raad RA, Rakheja R, et al.** Fluorodeoxyglucose positron emission tomography with computed tomography detects greater metabolic changes that are not represented by plain radiography for patients with osteonecrosis of the jaw. *J Oral Maxillofac Surg.* 2014 Oct; 72(10):1957–1965.

34. **Fleisher KE, Pham S, Raad RA, et al.** Does fluorodeoxyglucose positron emission tomography with computed tomography facilitate treatment of medication-related osteonecrosis of the jaw? *J Oral Maxillofac Surg.* 2015 Nov 6. pii: S0278-2391(15)01435-4. doi: 10.1016/j.joms.2015.10.025. Epub ahead of print.

35. **Aghaloo TL, Dry SM, Mallya S, et al.** Stage 0 osteonecrosis of the jaw in a patient on denosumab. *J Oral Maxillofac Surg.* 2014 Apr; 72(4):702–716.

36. **Farias DS, Zen Filho EV, de Oliveira TF, et al.** Clinical and image findings in bisphosphonate-related osteonecrosis of the jaws. *J Craniofac Surg.* 2013 Jul; 24(4):1248–1251.

37. **Fedele S, Porter SR, D'Aiuto F, et al.** Nonexposed variant of bisphosphonate-associated osteonecrosis of the jaw: a case series. *Am J Med.* 2010 Nov; 123(11):1060–1064.

4 Treatment and outcomes measures for antiresorptive drug-related osteonecrosis of the jaw

Oliver Ristow, Alberto Bedogni, Stefano Fedele

1 Introductory questions

In this chapter, four questions are raised and discussed:
- What are the real aims of treatment for antiresorptive drug-related osteonecrosis of the jaw (ARONJ)?
- What are relevant outcomes measures for the treatment of ARONJ?
- What is the impact of definition and staging for ARONJ?
- What therapeutic strategies exist for ARONJ?

2 Outcomes measures

Antiresorptive agents, including bisphosphonates and denosumab, have beneficial effects for the overwhelming majority of patients with osteoporosis, metastatic bone disease, and multiple myeloma, with significant reduction in skeletal-related events and an overall improvement in quality of life [1–7]. However, it has also been well established that a small subgroup of patients exposed to antiresorptive therapy can develop ARONJ, a potentially severe adverse side effect associated with pain, infection, dysfunction, and an overall impaired quality of life. Although a significant body of literature has been produced over the last decade, there remains little evidence-based guidance for clinicians with respect to most aspects of this disease. One particularly unclear aspect, and certainly one of the most controversial, is the therapy for ARONJ: there remains no robust evidence supporting any particular intervention in its management due to the lack of well designed randomized controlled trials. In particular, it is not known whether affected individuals should be offered symptomatic noncurative therapy such as infection and pain management with possibly minimally invasive debridement of superficial necrotic bone, or if potentially curative resective bone surgery should be attempted.

The topic is complex, as there is a portion of ARONJ patients that have minimal symptoms and relatively mild disease and may therefore benefit from minimally invasive management. In contrast, there are others with a painful, progressing disease that does not respond to symptomatic management and who therefore require more aggressive intervention. It is widely accepted that nonsurgical therapy aims to minimize symptoms and resolve infections rather than remove necrotic bone [8, 9], and one may argue that this should simply be considered an improvement of the patient's status and quality of life but cannot be labeled as successful curative management of necrotic bone disease. Indeed determinants of quality of life are not limited to absence of pain and infection, and therefore the lack of mucosal integrity, tooth loss, halitosis, and loss of sensation can still affect quality of life irrespective of the presence of pain and infection.

Furthermore, the underlying medical status of ARONJ-affected individuals should always be taken into account as many patients have incurable malignant disease, a short life expectancy, and poor performance status, which would automatically rule out the option of an aggressive surgical intervention. Yet, since the introduction of new potent anticancer therapies in the last decade (eg, antivascular endothelial growth factor (anti-VEGF), tyrosine kinase inhibitors, and more recently, mammalian target of rapamycin (m-TOR) inhibitors), overall survival curves have improved in many cancer types to an extent that the surgical therapy of ONJ should be no longer excluded "a priori" in metastatic cancer patients.

In addition to the lack of well-designed clinical studies on interventions, another major unclear aspect relates to the outcomes measures of ARONJ therapy. Many studies, for example, use long-term mucosal integrity ("mucosal healing") and no recurrence of bone exposure as the main outcome measure [10–16], although this has not been adequately validated, is controversial, and lacks in consistency and reproducibility. Furthermore, posttherapy follow-up periods in available studies vary from weeks to months, and therefore the endpoint for the collection of outcome measures also varies widely. Another unclear aspect of treatment outcomes is relevant to the concept of disease recurrence versus development of new sites of osteonecrosis, which in turn is related to the absence of clear radiological criteria to define the extent of the disease and necrotic bone.

Finally, very little is known regarding the potential use of patient-related outcome measures for ARONJ and of quality of life instruments used in assessing responses to therapy. This is of great importance especially in the context of cancer therapy aiming at ensuring a good quality of life in people living with incurable cancer, as management of ARONJ may similarly aim at minimizing patients' symptoms and infection and therefore improving quality of life rather than "curing" the osteonecrosis [8, 9, 17].

The topic is highly controversial and there remains no consensus and no clear guidance for clinicians. However, more recent studies have started to unravel some of the uncertainties related to ARONJ therapy. For example, when mucosal healing is adopted as a main outcomes measure, a current multivariate analysis showed lower recurrence rates for surgically treated ARONJ patients when compared with conservative nonsurgical treatment protocols [18, 19]. Thus, recently performed systematic reviews suggest that surgical treatment protocols can be superior to nonoperative management [20, 21].

However, as previously mentioned, these data simply refer to clinician-based assessment of mucosal healing and do not include any radiological or histological assessments to demonstrate the complete resection of diseased bone, and therefore the absence of bony abnormality underneath the mucosa. In addition, these results are limited by an embarrassing lack of consistent and validated patient-centered outcomes measures. There is an urgent need for future research to develop consistent outcomes measures that are both clinician and patient-centered. Quality of life instruments should represent an essential outcome measure in clinical studies of ARONJ therapy. The endpoints of outcome collection should also be long-term and standardized. Future studies should also consider the use of histological criteria so as to define complete resection of diseased bone (for surgical studies) and the adoption of radiological criteria so as to demonstrate the absence of bony abnormalities even in patients with complete mucosal healing and no notable symptoms, as previously suggested by some authors [22].

3   Impact of disease definition and staging on the outcomes of ARONJ treatment

Most available staging systems for osteonecrosis, including the widely used American Association of Oral and Maxillofacial Surgeons (AAOMS) system, classify staging and severity on the basis of clinical and radiographic findings. They also provide stage-related treatment recommendations [23]. However, clinical inspection and plain radiography are limited in their ability to identify the extent of necrotic bone disease compared with computed tomography (CT). A staging system that does not include accurate imaging of the affected bone is likely to lead to an incomplete and incorrect estimate of the extent of the disease, which in turn would lead to incorrect treatment recommendations. Bedogni et al have demonstrated that the AAOMS staging system does not correctly identify the extent of bony disease in ARONJ patients; they showed evidence of CT-proven diffuse bone disease in patients that were classified as having an early AAOMS stage (stage 0 and 1) (**Figs 4-1, 4-2**), and demonstrated localized/focal bone disease on CT in a significant number of patients classified as having a more advanced AAOMS stage (stage 2) [24]. These findings possibly explain the variability of responses to treatment reported for patients with AAOMS stage 1 and 2 disease, as this groups include individuals with heterogeneous extent, and therefore, severity of bone disease (focal and diffuse). Other limitations of the current AAOMS classification system, which can have an impact upon treatment outcomes, include: (1) neither the extent of the exposed bone nor its location are taken into account, (2) combined ARONJ symptoms are not considered and therefore cannot clearly be classified, (3) the underlying medical condition as well as the patient's status are not considered. Therefore, it is of great importance that studies on therapy success should not use retrospective but instead prospective study designs. It is a pitfall of retrospective studies conducted with questionnaires without oral investigations to miss early stages with exposed bone that are not accompanied by infection or pain. Due to the fact that these 'silent' ARONJ stages are a frequent finding, a significant number of cases are not recorded in retrospective studies. Also, it has been increasingly discussed that superficial clinical signs (as commonly used for most staging systems) may not show the true extent of bony disease, therefore under- or overestimating the prognosis, leading to misinterpretations and repercussion on therapeutic decisions [19, 24].

The definition of ARONJ is another crucial aspect in the critical assessment of the outcomes of ARONJ therapy. Earlier definitions of ARONJ involved the presence of exposed jaw bone for a period of at least 8 weeks [25–27]. However, recent data suggests that these traditional definitions excluded patients that presented with a nonexposed variant of the condition. Fedele et al demonstrated that the use of the traditional definition could result in up to 25% of ARONJ patients remaining undiagnosed [28]. Although the recently revised AAOMS classification of ARONJ includes patients presenting with mucosal sinus tracts and no obvious bone exposure, the ARONJ definition was paradoxically not amended and therefore individuals with the nonexposed

variant remained undiagnosed by AAOMS criteria. The above inconsistencies in disease staging and differences in disease definition have most likely led to inclusion into clinical studies and retrospective analyses of highly heterogeneous groups of patients. Similarly, there has been heterogeneity in assessing responses to therapy and disease status. For example, an ARONJ patient with development of fistula tract and, paradoxically, a mandibular fracture after treatment would be classified to be in remission because of the absence of necrotic bone exposure. It is not unrealistic to suggest that these inconsistencies and limitations have led to major differences in treatment outcomes among published studies.

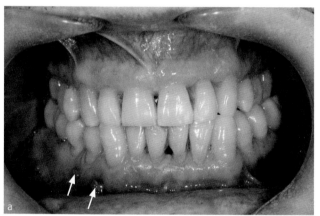
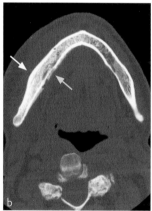

Fig 4-1a–b　Intraoral view of an ARONJ patient presenting with two nonsuppurating mucosal fistulas at the level of the right mandibular body (Stage 1 AAOMS, 2014) (white arrows) (**a**). The patient's axial CT scan showing involvement of the entire right mandibular body with bone condensation (white arrow) and all-embracing periosteal osteoblastic reaction (yellow arrow) (**b**).

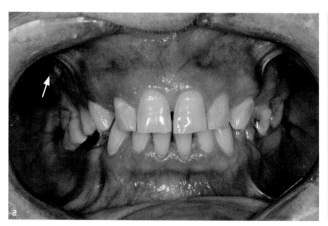
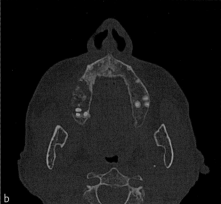

Fig 4-2a–b　Intraoral view of an ARONJ patient presenting with two suppurating mucosal fistulas at the posterior aspect of the right maxilla (Stage 2 AAOMS, 2014) (white arrow) (**a**). The patient's axial CT scan showing bone condensation of the entire maxilla and bone sequestra formation at the level of the molar region (**b**).

4   Therapeutic strategies

There remains no consensus regarding the optimal management of patients with ARONJ. When mucosal healing is the primary aim of the treatment, a number of studies have suggested that surgery should represent the first line of therapy, especially when clear identification of disease margins allows complete resection of the necrotic bone [12, 29–31]. Indeed Hoff et al [10] and Nicolatou-Galitis et al [11] reported conservative nonsurgical management to be associated with complete mucosal healing in only 23% and 14.9% of patients respectively, notably after a median of 8 months of therapy. It is also worth mentioning that some of the patients that showed complete healing after nonoperative management had nonexposed stage 0 ARONJ [23, 27]. Nevertheless, other authors have emphasized that ARONJ treatment should focus on pain and infection control, especially in individuals with short-life expectancy and poor performance status and who may experience significant postoperative complications [32, 33]. They suggest that persistence of necrotic bone underneath the mucosal surface could be compatible with good quality of life, especially when secondary infections are prevented and pain is controlled, and when there is little convincing evidence that a nonoperative approach would cause progression of ARONJ. Those in favor of surgical intervention, however, suggest that nonoperative measures cannot "cure" ARONJ and that the persistence of bone exposure and associated recurrent infections can also affect the delivery of future cancer chemotherapy and antiresorptive therapy [34, 35]. They highlight that, historically, surgical therapy has been central to the treatment of chronic necrotic tissue, regardless of the cause.

Necrosis has often been approached with surgical removal as a main part of the treatment algorithm since tissue necrosis is irreversible and will continue to exist as a complex chronic wound prone to complications (eg, secondary infection) [12, 36]. With respect to ARONJ, the surgical removal of necrotic bone tissue has been approached with either minimally invasive surgical debridement or resective surgery, which have been associated with a variety of success rates [19, 36, 37]. The primary goal always ought to be to resect as much as necessary and as less as possible [38]. Debridement represents a cautious and empirical suboptimal approach that reduces but cannot completely eliminate necrotic bone [12, 19]. On the contrary, resection is planned with accurate preoperative imaging (eg, CT) and carried out so as to obtain healthy bone margin. Therefore marginal, segmental, or even subtotal to total resection are likely to be associated with complete removal of necrotic bone tissue (**Figs 4-3, 4-4**).

However, the challenge of surgical treatment is that the exact margins of ARONJ are difficult to determine, thus a clear demarcation of the necrotic bone is difficult if not impossible to achieve [25, 39]. The complete removal of necrotic bone is of crucial importance as otherwise there is the risk of disease recurrence or progression [12, 18].

The other challenge of surgical treatment is the lack of standardization of surgical procedures, as these depend on the ability and experience of the surgeon and are difficult to compare and reproduce. One of the most commonly adopted parameters is the intraoperative impression of the surgeon [40, 41]. Surgical debridement and resection in ARONJ therapy is commonly performed until the bone appears to be "normal" in structure, color, and texture, with bleeding being widely accepted to be a sign of viable bone [38]. The exposed bone in ARONJ lesions commonly shows a darker and yellowish color, as well as increased porosity, as compared to healthy bone. However, the necrotic bone of ARONJ is commonly surrounded by sclerotic bone areas, which are harder and can present with various degrees of vascularization ranging from poorly to highly inflamed and hypervascularized tissue [22, 42]. Therefore, using bone bleeding for guidance can be misleading. Furthermore, it has been shown that bone bleeding does not always correlate with the histological findings of vital unaffected bone [30]. In conclusion, bleeding cannot be used as an absolute parameter to determine the extent or the margins of surgery in ARONJ patients [30, 39, 43].

The use of imaging techniques (eg, CT and MRI) has been suggested to distinguish between healthy and diseased bone tissue preoperatively, with various degrees of success [44–46]. Other authors successfully implemented the use of histology to confirm the appropriateness of bone resection and the presence of healthy bone margins, as they were determined preoperatively on the basis of CT and MRI [14].

An alternative strategy to distinguish between viable and necrotic bone is the use of bone fluorescence [30, 39, 43, 47, 48]. Tetracycline and its derivates possess fluorescence properties [49], which under appropriate excitation light (525–540 nm) can show visible greenish fluorescence [50]. Due to its affinity to calcium, tetracyclines are incorporated into bone in particular in areas of high bone turn-over [51]. Viable normal bone shows a green fluorescence that can be visualized intraoperatively by using a VELscope fluorescence lamp (eg, LED Dental, White Rock, British Columbia, Canada), a certified medical device originally developed for the detection of mucosal tissue abnormalities [29, 30, 39, 43, 47]. In contrast, necrotic bone shows no or only pale fluorescence.

Recent reports suggest that the VELscope system may induce an auto-fluorescence of vital but not of necrotic bone (**Figs 4-5, 4-6**) without tetracycline bone labeling leading to similar bone fluorescence of tetracycline-exposed tissue [52].

As a consequence, fluorescence allows the surgeon to identify the margin between viable and necrotic bone and remove the diseased bone until the remaining bone is fluorescing under the VELscope light. Of note, reddish fluorescence is considered as bacterial colonization of the bone. These areas should be further removed even if green bone fluorescence is present. Due to the fact that this technique is easy to apply, reproducible, and does not rely on the subjective impression of the surgeon, it is an important milestone towards a standardization of the surgical ARONJ therapy auguring an improvement of the treatment. Indeed, this technique will not avoid significant resection if necessary, but it will standardize surgical practice.

Still, there might not be enough data to draw final conclusions regarding the optimal treatment protocol, especially as there is hardly any data on how to manage ARONJ cases

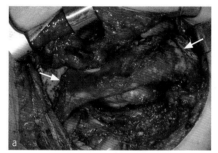
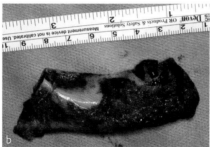
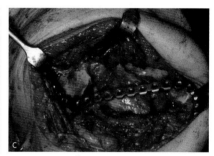

Fig 4-3a–c Resection and mandibulectomy for an ARONJ patient.
a Intraoperative view of a typical segmental resection of the mandible in an ARONJ patient. The margins of bone resection as planned on CT and MRI are outlined (white arrows).
b Intraoperative view of the surgical specimen.
c Intraoperative view of the reconstruction of the lateral defect following mandibulectomy. A locking reconstruction plate 2.4 was used to span the defect and to restore mandibular continuity. Single-layer mucosal closure of the defect was achieved without tension.

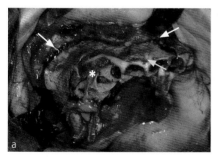
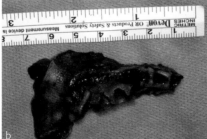
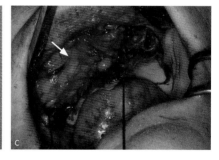

Fig 4-4a–c Resection and maxillectomy for an ARONJ patient.
a Intraoperative view showing a standard lower maxillectomy procedure. The margins of bone resection, as planned on CT and MRI are outlined (white arrows). The initially exposed and necrotic bone in the oral cavity is obvious (white asterisk), as compared with the adjacent nonexposed necrotic/inflamed bone that can be seen following mucosal incision (yellow arrow).
b Intraoperative view of the surgical specimen.
c Intraoperative view of the reconstruction of the lower maxillectomy defect. Double-layer closure of the defect was warranted to seal the orosinonasal communication, using Bichat's buccal fat pad (white arrow) and mucosal advancement flaps.

under denosumab in which nonoperative treatment protocols might play a different role due to the much shorter half-life. The clinical decision-making will always be based on individual risk assessment especially as most of the patients suffering from ARONJ have multiple underlying diseases. This process requires knowledge about the chances and limitations of the treatment options. Unfortunately, the vast majority of clinical trials of interventions for ARONJ are characterized by poor methodology, lack of control arm, and missing randomization. It is therefore difficult to ultimately support either nonoperative strategies or surgical procedures for either stage. Indeed, it is of paramount importance that future research focuses on high-quality randomized and controlled trials, possibly comparing surgical versus nonoperative therapy. It is also worth investigating the effects of surgical debridement versus resective procedures.

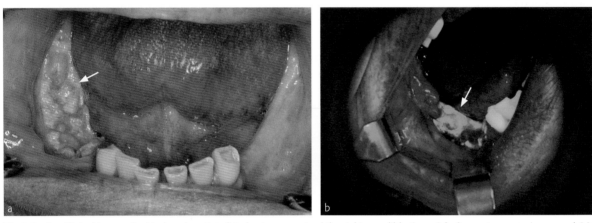

Fig 4-5a–b   Clinical image of a bisphosphonate-related osteonecrosis of the right mandible (arrow) before osteonecrosis removal (**a**). The corresponding field of view using the VELscope Vx system (**b**). Note that necrotic bone areas showed no or only very pale autofluorescence (arrow).

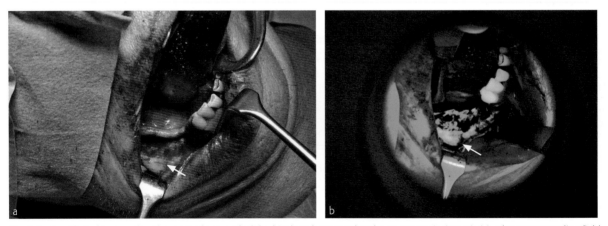

Fig 4-6a–b   Clinical image after the surgical removal of the bisphosphonate-related osteonecrosis (arrow) (**a**). The corresponding field of view using the VELscope Vx system without tetracycline labeling (**b**). Note that the bone areas showed a bright auto-fluorescence after removal of the osteonecrosis (arrow).

5 Conclusion

Since the topic is highly controversial and there still remains no consensus, there is an urgent need for future research to develop consistent outcomes measures that should be both clinician and patient-centered (eg, quality of life instruments). Great effort should be taken to adapt disease staging and disease definition to achieve homogenous study groups for future evidence-based high-quality data. Although surgical intervention seems to be a superior alternative, it is only through randomized and controlled trials that robust data can be produced in order to develop genuine recommendations for future ARONJ therapy guidelines.

6 References

1. **Berenson JR, Lichtenstein A, Porter L, et al.** Efficacy of pamidronate in reducing skeletal events in patients with advanced multiple myeloma. Myeloma Aredia Study Group. *N Engl J Med.* 1996 Feb; 334(8):488–493.

2. **Black DM, Cummings SR, Karpf DB, et al.** Randomised trial of effect of alendronate on risk of fracture in women with existing vertebral fractures. Fracture Intervention Trial Research Group. *Lancet.* 1996 Dec; 348(9041):1535–1541.

3. **Black DM, Delmas PD, Eastell R, et al.** Once-yearly zoledronic acid for treatment of postmenopausal osteoporosis. *N Engl J Med.* 2007 May; 356(18):1809–1822.

4. **Black DM, Schwartz AV, Ensrud KE, et al.** Effects of continuing or stopping alendronate after 5 years of treatment: the Fracture Intervention Trial Long-term Extension (FLEX): a randomized trial. *Jama.* 2006 Dec; 296(24):2927–2938.

5. **Corso A, Varettoni M, Zappasodi P, et al.** A different schedule of zoledronic acid can reduce the risk of the osteonecrosis of the jaw in patients with multiple myeloma. *Leukemia.* 2007 Jul; 21(7):1545–1548.

6. **Cummings SR, San Martin J, McClung MR, et al.** Denosumab for prevention of fractures in postmenopausal women with osteoporosis. *N Engl J Med.* 2009 Aug; 361(8):756–765.

7. **Morgan GJ, Davies FE, Gregory WM, et al.** First-line treatment with zoledronic acid as compared with clodronic acid in multiple myeloma (MRC Myeloma IX): a randomised controlled trial. *Lancet.* 2010 Dec; 376(9757):1989–1999.

8. **Badros A, Terpos E, Katodritou E, et al.** Natural history of osteonecrosis of the jaw in patients with multiple myeloma. *J Clin Oncol.* 2008 Dec; 26(36):5904–5909.

9. **Van den Wyngaert T, Claeys T, Huizing MT, et al.** Initial experience with conservative treatment in cancer patients with osteonecrosis of the jaw (ONJ) and predictors of outcome. *Ann Oncol.* 2009 Feb; 20(2):331–336.

10. **Hoff AO, Toth BB, Altundag K, et al.** Frequency and risk factors associated with osteonecrosis of the jaw in cancer patients treated with intravenous bisphosphonates. *J Bone Miner Res.* 2008 Jun; 23(6):826–836.

11. **Nicolatou-Galitis O, Papadopoulou E, Sarri T, et al.** Osteonecrosis of the jaw in oncology patients treated with bisphosphonates: prospective experience of a dental oncology referral center. *Oral Surg Oral Med Oral Pathol Oral Radiol Endod.* 2011 Aug; 112(2):195–202.

12. **Carlson ER, Basile JD.** The role of surgical resection in the management of bisphosphonate-related osteonecrosis of the jaws. *J Oral Maxillofac Surg.* 2009 May; 67(5 Suppl):S85–95.

13. **Stockmann P, Vairaktaris E, Wehrhan F, et al.** Osteotomy and primary wound closure in bisphosphonate-associated osteonecrosis of the jaw: a prospective clinical study with 12 months follow-up. *Support Care Cancer.* 2010 Apr; 18(4):449–460.

14. **Bedogni A, Saia G, Bettini G, et al.** Long-term outcomes of surgical resection of the jaws in cancer patients with bisphosphonate-related osteonecrosis. *Oral Oncol.* 2011 May; 47(5):420–424.

15. **Schubert M, Klatte I, Linek W, et al.** The saxon bisphosphonate register—therapy and prevention of bisphosphonate-related osteonecrosis of the jaws. *Oral Oncol.* 2012 Apr; 48(4):349–354.

16. **Jacobsen C, Metzler P, Obwegeser JA, et al.** Osteopathology of the jaw associated with bone resorption inhibitors: what have we learned in the last 8 years? *Swiss Med Wkly.* 2012; 142:w13605.

17. **Kyrgidis A, Triaridis S, Kontos K, et al.** Quality of life in breast cancer patients with bisphosphonate-related osteonecrosis of the jaws and patients with head and neck cancer: a comparative study using the EORTC QLQ-C30 and QLQ-HN35 questionnaires. *Anticancer Res.* 2012 Aug; 32(8):3527–3534.

18. **Mucke T, Koschinski J, Deppe H, et al.** Outcome of treatment and parameters influencing recurrence in patients with bisphosphonate-related osteonecrosis of the jaws. *J Cancer Res Clin Oncol.* 2011 May; 137(5):907–913.

19. **Graziani F, Vescovi P, Campisi G, et al.** Resective surgical approach shows a high performance in the management of advanced cases of bisphosphonate-related osteonecrosis of the jaws: a retrospective survey of 347 cases. *J Oral Maxillofac Surg.* 2012 Nov; 70(11):2501–2507.

20. **Fliefel R, Troltzsch M, Kuhnisch J, et al.** Treatment strategies and outcomes of bisphosphonate-related osteonecrosis of the jaw (BRONJ) with characterization of patients: a systematic review. *Int J Oral Maxillofac Surg.* 2015 May; 44(5):568–585.

21. **Rupel K, Ottaviani G, Gobbo M, et al.** A systematic review of therapeutical approaches in bisphosphonates-related osteonecrosis of the jaw (BRONJ). *Oral Oncol.* 2014 Nov; 50(11):1049–1057.

22. **Bedogni A, Blandamura S, Lokmic Z, et al.** Bisphosphonate-associated jawbone osteonecrosis: a correlation between imaging techniques and histopathology. *Oral Surg Oral Med Oral Pathol Oral Radiol Endod.* 2008 Mar; 105(3):358–364.

23. **Ruggiero SL, Dodson TB, Fantasia J, et al.** American Association of Oral and Maxillofacial Surgeons position paper on medication-related osteonecrosis of the jaw—2014 update. *J Oral Maxillofac Surg.* 2014 Oct; 72(10):1938–1956. Epub 5/5/2014.

24. **Bedogni A, Fedele S, Bedogni G, et al.** Staging of osteonecrosis of the jaw requires computed tomography for accurate definition of the extent of bony disease. *Br J Oral Maxillofac Surg.* 2014 Sep; 52(7):603–608.

25. **Khosla S, Burr D, Cauley J, et al.** Bisphosphonate-associated osteonecrosis of the jaw: report of a task force of the American Society for Bone and Mineral Research. *J Bone Miner Res.* 2007 Oct; 22(10):1479–1491.

26. **American Association of Oral and Maxillofacial Surgeons.** Position paper on bisphosphonate-related osteonecrosis of the jaws. *J Oral Maxillofac Surg.* 2007 Mar; 65(3):369–376.

27. **Ruggiero SL, Dodson TB, Assael LA, et al.** American Association of Oral and Maxillofacial Surgeons position paper on bisphosphonate-related osteonecrosis of the jaws—2009 update. *J Oral Maxillofac Surg.* 2009 May; 67(5 Suppl):S2–12.

28. **Fedele S, Bedogni G, Scoletta M, et al.** Up to a quarter of patients with osteonecrosis of the jaw associated with antiresorptive agents remain undiagnosed. *Br J Oral Maxillofac Surg.* 2015 Jan; 53(1):13–17.

29. **Assaf AT, Zrnc TA, Riecke B, et al.** Intraoperative efficiency of fluorescence imaging by Visually Enhanced Lesion Scope (VELscope) in patients with bisphosphonate related osteonecrosis of the jaw (BRONJ). *J Craniomaxillofac Surg.* 2014 Jul; 42(5):e157–164. Epub 9/4/2013.

30. **Pautke C, Bauer F, Otto S, et al.** Fluorescence-guided bone resection in bisphosphonate-related osteonecrosis of the jaws: first clinical results of a prospective pilot study. *J Oral Maxillofac Surg.* 2011 Jan; 69(1):84–91.

31. **Vescovi P, Manfredi M, Merigo E, et al.** Early surgical approach preferable to medical therapy for bisphosphonate-related osteonecrosis of the jaws. *J Oral Maxillofac Surg.* 2008 Apr; 66(4):831–832.

32. **Khan AA, Morrison A, Hanley DA, et al.** Diagnosis and management of osteonecrosis of the jaw: a systematic review and international consensus. *J Bone Miner Res.* 2015 Jan; 30(1):3–23.

33. **Bodem JP, Kargus S, Eckstein S, et al.** Incidence of bisphosphonate-related osteonecrosis of the jaw in high-risk patients undergoing surgical tooth extraction. *J Craniomaxillofac Surg.* 2015 May; 43(4):510–514. Epub 3/9/2015.

34. **Then C, Horauf N, Otto S, et al.** Incidence and risk factors of bisphosphonate-related osteonecrosis of the jaw in multiple myeloma patients having undergone autologous stem cell transplantation. *Onkologie.* 2012; 35(11):658–664.

35. **Otto S, Schreyer C, Hafner S, et al.** Bisphosphonate-related osteonecrosis of the jaws—characteristics, risk factors, clinical features, localization and impact on oncological treatment. *J Craniomaxillofac Surg.* 2012 Jun; 40(4):303–309.

36. **Carlson ER.** Management of antiresorptive osteonecrosis of the jaws with primary surgical resection. *J Oral Maxillofac Surg.* 2014 Apr; 72(4):655–657.

37. **Jabbour Z, El-Hakim M, Mesbah-Ardakani P, et al.** The outcomes of conservative and surgical treatment of stage 2 bisphosphonate-related osteonecrosis of the jaws: a case series. *Int J Oral Maxillofac Surg.* 2012 Nov; 41(11):1404–1409.

38. **Ristow O, Otto S, Troeltzsch M, et al.** Treatment perspectives for medication-related osteonecrosis of the jaw (MRONJ). *J Craniomaxillofac Surg.* 2015 Mar; 43(2):290–293. Epub 11/22/2014.

39. **Pautke C, Bauer F, Tischer T, et al.** Fluorescence-guided bone resection in bisphosphonate-associated osteonecrosis of the jaws. *J Oral Maxillofac Surg.* 2009 Mar; 67(3):471–476.

40. **Guggenberger R, Fischer DR, Metzler P, et al.** Bisphosphonate-induced osteonecrosis of the jaw: comparison of disease extent on contrast-enhanced MR imaging, [18F] fluoride PET/CT, and conebeam CT imaging. *AJNR Am J Neuroradiol.* 2013 Jun-Jul; 34(6):1242–1247.

41. **Otto S.** *Medication-Related Osteonecrosis of the Jaws.* Berlin Heidelberg: Springer; 2015.

42. **Otto S, Baumann S, Ehrenfeld M, et al.** Successful surgical management of osteonecrosis of the jaw due to RANK-ligand inhibitor treatment using fluorescence guided bone resection. *J Craniomaxillofac Surg.* 2013 Oct; 41(7):694–698.

43. **Pautke C, Bauer F, Bissinger O, et al.** Tetracycline bone fluorescence: a valuable marker for osteonecrosis characterization and therapy. *J Oral Maxillofac Surg.* 2010 Jan; 68(1):125–129.

44. **Stockmann P, Hinkmann FM, Lell MM, et al.** Panoramic radiograph, computed tomography or magnetic resonance imaging. Which imaging technique should be preferred in bisphosphonate-associated osteonecrosis of the jaw? A prospective clinical study. *Clin Oral Investig.* 2010 Jun; 14(3):311–317.

45. **Wilde F, Heufelder M, Winter K, et al.** The role of surgical therapy in the management of intravenous bisphosphonates-related osteonecrosis of the jaw. *Oral Surg Oral Med Oral Pathol Oral Radiol Endod.* 2011 Feb; 111(2):153–163.

46. **Voss PJ, Joshi Oshero J, Kovalova-Muller A, et al.** Surgical treatment of bisphosphonate-associated osteonecrosis of the jaw: technical report and follow up of 21 patients. *J Craniomaxillofac Surg.* 2012 Dec; 40(8):719–725.

47. **Pautke C, Tischer T, Neff A, et al.** In vivo tetracycline labeling of bone: an intraoperative aid in the surgical therapy of osteoradionecrosis of the mandible. *Oral Surg Oral Med Oral Pathol Oral Radiol Endod.* 2006 Dec; 102(6):e10–13.

48. **Fleisher KE, Doty S, Kottal S, et al.** Tetracycline-guided debridement and cone beam computed tomography for the treatment of bisphosphonate-related osteonecrosis of the jaw: a technical note. *J Oral Maxillofac Surg.* 2008 Dec; 66(12):2646–2653.

49. **Harris WH.** A microscopic method of determining rates of bone growth. *Nature.* 1960 Dec; 188:1038–1039.

50. **Pautke C, Vogt S, Kreutzer K, et al.** Characterization of eight different tetracyclines: advances in fluorescence bone labeling. *J Anat.* 2010 Jul; 217(1):76–82.

51. **Rauch F, Travers R, Glorieux FH.** Intracortical remodeling during human bone development—a histomorphometric study. *Bone.* 2007 Feb; 40(2):274–280.

52. **Ristow O, Pautke C.** Auto-fluorescence of the bone and its use for delineation of bone necrosis. *Int J Oral Maxillofac Surg.* 2014 Nov; 43(11):1391–1393. Epub 8/12/2014.

5 Risk factors for antiresorptive drug-related osteonecrosis of the jaw

Robert E Marx

1 Introductory questions

In this chapter, four questions are raised and discussed:

- What are the real risk factors for antiresorptive drug-related osteonecrosis of the jaw (ARONJ)?
- What are the initiation factors for ARONJ?
- Where are the vulnerable sites?
- What are the relevant comorbidities?

2 Definition

A risk factor is defined as a gene, disease, drug, habit, or other factor that predisposes an individual to developing a medical condition with or without other influences. Examples of such risk factors include the BRCA-1 gene, which predisposes and results in some women developing breast cancer, or cigarette smoking, which causes both oral pharyngeal and lung cancers without any other influences. Unfortunately, the current specialty association taskforce papers have not adhered to such a direct link and have included as risk factors a myriad of coincidental conditions that have not in the past, nor presently, independently resulted in osteonecrosis of the jaws (ONJ) [1, 2]. These taskforce papers, and even some medical publications, have advanced obesity, female gender, smoking, tori, and tooth extraction as ONJ risk factors [3, 4, 5]. Clearly none of these, nor the many more they list, result in long standing exposed bone in the jaws by themselves. Overweight people do not develop ONJ simply from over-eating, and thousands of teeth are taken out every day without causing ONJ unless a true risk factor such as previous radiation therapy, a history of bisphosphonate (BP) intake, or reactive activator of nuclear kappa B ligand (RANKL) inhibitor use has been present. Also, being a woman clearly does not predispose someone to ONJ without one of the true risk factors being present.

The following then is a more straightforward identification of scientifically correct risk factors. Also provided is a stratification of previously incorrectly labeled risk factors into initiating factors, vulnerable sites, and comorbidities.

3 Risk factors

The primary risk factor for ARONJ is the drug itself. Today, four drugs classifications have provided sufficient evidence and a track record of causing ONJ to be considered true risk factors:

- Bisphosphonates, due to their mechanism of apoptosis (killing) of osteoclasts mostly at the bone resorption site [6] (**Figs 5-1, 5-2**) and to a lesser degree on osteoclastic precursors in bone marrow as well as a mild antiangiogenic effect on small blood vessels [7] (eg, alendronate, zoledronate)
- Reactive activator of nuclear kappa B ligand (RANKL) inhibitors, due to their impairment as well as killing of adult osteoclasts as well as precursors at all stages of osteoclast development [8] (eg, denosumab)
- Potent antiangiogenic drugs, due to their inhibition of vascular endothelial growth factor (VEGF), which results in an avascular bone necrosis [9] (eg, bevacizumab)
- Potent tyrosine kinase (TRK) inhibitors, due to their irreversible inhibition of several cell membrane-intracellular transcription factor relationships resulting in cellular death [10] (eg, sunitinib).

In addition, factors such as dosage, potency, and administration should also be considered risk factors.

3.1   Dose

It is well known that for almost every pharmaceutical drug, from aspirin to digitalis, increased dosing results in a more profound effect and a greater number and severity of complications. Today, alendronate is the cause of 95% of all oral BP-induced osteonecrosis compared with residronate (3%) or ibandronate (1%). This is due to its recommended dose of 70 mg/week as compared with residronate at 35 mg/week and ibandronate 150 mg/month, which equates to 35 mg/week. Similarly, denosumab at 120 mg subcutaneously monthly for metastatic cancer control and control of hypercalcemia produces a greater number of cases and a greater severity of ONJ than denosumab at 60 mg subcutaneously every 6 months for osteoporosis (**Figs 5-3, 5-4**).

3.2   Potency

The potency of a drug is its biologic effect per dose weight. **Table 5-1** lists the relative potencies of the more commonly administered BPs. One can see that alendronate and zoledronate have the greatest measured potency. It is these two drugs that account for the vast majority of ARONJ cases. Since the two marketed denosumab preparations are the same drug, their potency is the same, identifying that the focus of their relative risk is related to the vast differences in their dose and frequency of administration.

3.3   Route of administration

All publications and taskforce position papers agree that intravenous BPs cause a greater number of cases and a more severe and extensive ONJ than that caused by oral BPs [1, 2, 11, 12]. This is due to the poor gut absorption of oral BPs (0.64%) resulting in a 140 times greater bio-availability from the intravenous route. The RANKL inhibitors are all administered subcutaneously, once again focusing their risk more on dose and frequency.

3.4   Frequency of administration

Osteoclast precursors in bone marrow, as well as in the human body in general, have a remarkable recovery and repopulation ability. Consecutive exposures to toxins spaced out over long intervals are better tolerated than consecutive exposures with short interval periods. This may explain to some degree the reduced incidence of ONJ from the once monthly dosing of ibandronate as compared to the once weekly dosing of residronate and alendronate. This relationship to frequency of administration has also been recognized by many clinical oncologists, who are now administering IV zoledronate at every 3 or 6 months, which is off-label from the manufacturer's own advice of every 3 weeks to a month. Such a reduction in the frequency of administration has resulted in an observed reduction in the number and severity of cases.

3.5   Half-life in bone

The terminal half-life of BPs has been measured at 11.2 years [13]. This is due to a strong affinity and irreversible binding to hydroxyapatite crystals in bone. Denosumab does not bind to bone but is metabolized in either the liver or kidney by the CYP450 enzyme with a published half-life of 26 days [8]. Clinically, this makes denosumab-induced ARONJ more straightforward to treat.

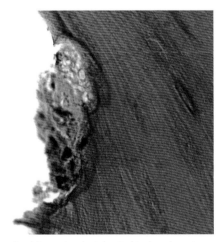

Fig 5-1   Initial phase of a dying osteoclast due to bisphosphonate ingestion. The nuclei are disrupted and there is free chromatin in the cytoplasm.

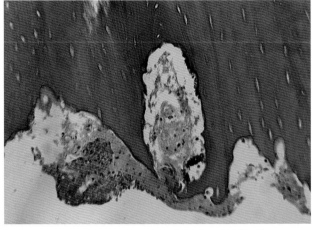

Fig 5-2   Late phase of a dying osteoclast due to bisphosphonate ingestion. The cell is now ballooned up and the nuclei are gone.

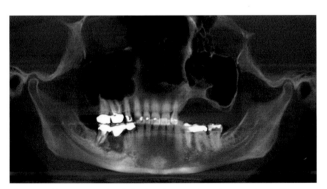

Fig 5-3 Osteonecrosis of the jaw in a patient that received 60 mg of denosumab subcutaneously every 6 months for 3 years.

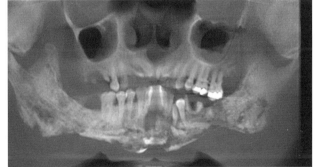

Fig 5-4 A more extensive osteonecrosis of the jaw in a patient that received 120 mg of denosumab subcutaneously monthly for 6 months.

Bisphosphonate	Potency
Etidronate	1
Tiludronate	50
Clodronate	500
Residronate	1,000
Ibandronate	1,000
Alendronate	5,000
Pamidronate	5,000
Zoledronate	10,000

Table 5-1 The relative potencies of bisphosphonates.

4   Initiation factors for osteonecrosis of the jaw

The removal of teeth or the existence of hyperocclusion or significant periodontal inflammation have been shown to be initiation factors for ONJ.

4.1   Tooth removal

Tooth removal is the initiator in up to 62% of ONJ cases (**Fig 5-5**) [12, 14]. This is due to the normal enhanced bone remolding rate of alveolar bone as compared to other bones as well as the greatly enhanced requirement for bone remodeling and regeneration required in a healing extraction socket.

4.2   Hyperocclusion

Although not previously well recognized, excessive occlusal forces initiate ONJ cases by requiring a greater rate and degree of remodeling in the alveolar bone [15]. Such occlusal overloading in BP and denosumab patients strongly correlate to a higher incidence seen in the molar areas in both jaws as well as the lingual balcony of the mandible, which is the focal point of axial loading during molar occlusion (**Fig 5-6**) [15].

4.3   Significant periodontal inflammation or surgery

Ongoing significant periodontal inflammation has been associated with developing ONJ in patients taking BPs [16]. This is due to the further increased alveolar bone remolding rate stimulated by the inflammatory process (**Fig 5-7**).

4.4   Surgery in alveolar bone

Surgeries in the alveolar bone other than tooth removal also increase the requirement for bone remodeling and renewal, which often cannot be met if osteoclastic function is impaired by a BP or denosumab (**Fig 5-8**).

4.5   Spontaneous ARONJ

Despite the above factors, about 25% of ARONJ cases occur without any identifiable initiating event (**Fig 5-9**) [14]. These cases are then directly related to the drug, its use, its potency, and its route and frequency of administration.

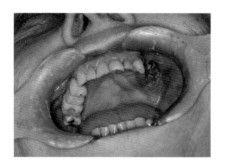

Fig 5-5   Maxillary ARONJ initiated by the extraction of posterior teeth.

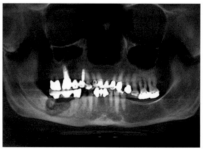

Fig 5-6   Hyperocclusion initiated this ARONJ in a patient that received alendronate for 4 years.

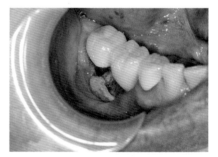

Fig 5-7   Chronic periodontal inflammation significantly contributed to this ARONJ.

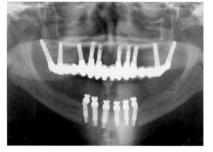

Fig 5-8   Dental implant surgery initiated this ARONJ of the mandible in a patient that had received alendronate for 5.5 years.

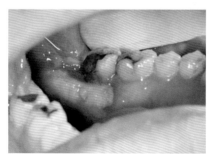

Fig 5-9   Spontaneously exposed bone representing ARONJ caused by using alendronate 70 mg/week for 5 years.

5 Vulnerable sites

Areas such as alveolar bone, the mandible, tori, and the midshaft of the femur can all be considered vulnerable sites for ARONJ.

5.1 Alveolar bone

In general, alveolar bone in either the mandible or maxilla represents the most vulnerable site, and with the exception of tori, all ARONJ cases that fit the numerous taskforce definitions of exposed bone start in alveolar bone [1, 2, 12, 14, 15]. This is due to the much greater requirement and rate of bone remodeling from normal as well as traumatic occlusion, and occasionally, denture wearing focused on the alveolar bone (**Fig 5-10**). Even ARONJ cases that arise spontaneously do so within alveolar bone.

5.2 Mandible greater than maxilla

Most large series identify a 2 to 1 predilection for ARONJ to occur in the mandible as compared with the maxilla [1, 11, 12, 14, 15].

5.3 Tori

Tori represents a truly vulnerable site rather than a risk factor (**Fig 5-11**). Because the bony surface of the tori continually remodels, it is affected by drugs that impair osteoclast mediated remodeling. Adding to this is the thin mucosa overlying tori [12, 15].

5.4 The midshaft (diaphysis) of the femur

Atypical subtrochanteric midshaft fractures of the femur have been linked to BP use in numerous publications (**Fig 5-12**) [17, 18, 19]. After alveolar bone in the mandible and maxilla, this area has the greatest requirement for remodeling resulting in such fractures. As one walks or runs, the femur, the longest bone in the skeleton, bends slightly at its midshaft. This bending moment requires bone remodeling, which BPs and denosumab prevent, resulting in a brittleness that promotes the many fractures that have been observed and reported.

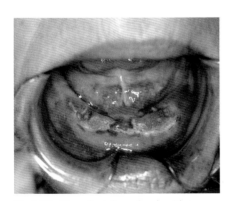

Fig 5-10 The edentulous alveolar ridge, a vulnerable site, which developed this spontaneous ARONJ.

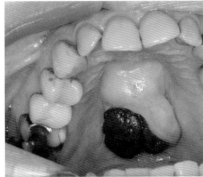

Fig 5-11 ARONJ in a maxillary torus, which represents a spontaneous ARONJ, and the torus is also a vulnerable site.

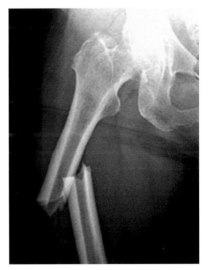

Fig 5-12 A spontaneous midshaft fracture of the femur caused by using alendronate for 8 years.

6   Comorbidities

Comorbidities do not cause a disease by themselves but may make it occur sooner and/or become more severe. There are numerous comorbidities. An incomplete list of those previously published as risk factors are as follows [19]:

- Smoking
- Diabetes
- Anemia
- Chemotherapy
- Cancer
- Corticosteroids
- Immune based diseases
  - Systemic lupus
  - Rheumatoid arthritis
- Dehydration
- Obesity.

7   Conclusion

Over the past decade, numerous potential risk factors for ARONJ have been proposed. However, many of these should instead be considered as initiating factors, vulnerable sites, or comorbidities. True risk factors include the actual drug or drugs provided to the patient, as well as the additional factors of dosage, potency, and route and frequency of administration. This chapter has aimed to clarify these issues based on exact science and the clinical experience of more than 500 cases.

8   References

1. **Ruggiero SL, Dodson TB, Fantasia J, et al.** American Association of Oral and Maxillofacial Surgeons position paper on medication-related osteonecrosis of the jaw—2014 update. *J Oral Maxillofac Surg.* 2014 Oct; 72(10):1938–1956.
2. **Khosla S, Burr D, Cauley J, et al.** Bisphosphonate-associated osteonecrosis of the jaw: report of a task force of the American Society for Bone and Mineral Research. *J Bone Miner Res.* 2007 Oct; 22(10):1479–1491.
3. **Wessel JH, Dodson TB, Zavras AI.** Zoledronate, smoking, and obesity are strong risk factors for osteonecrosis of the jaw: a case-control study. *J Oral Maxillofac Surg.* 2008 Apr; 66(4):625–631.
4. **Ruggiero S, Gralow J, Marx RE, et al.** Practical guidelines for the prevention, diagnosis, and treatment of osteonecrosis of the jaw in patients with cancer. *J Oncol Pract.* 2006 Jan; 2(1):7–14.
5. **Glick M.** Closing in on the Puzzle of ONJ. *J Am Dent Assoc.* 2008 Jan; 139(1):12, 14–15.
6. **Rogers MJ, Gordon S, Benford HL, et al.** Cellular and molecular mechanisms of action of bisphosphonates. *Cancer.* 2000 Jun 15; 88(12 Suppl):S2961–2978.
7. **Wood J, Bonjean K, Ruetz S, et al.** Novel antiangiogenic effects of the bisphosphonate compound zoledronic acid. *J Pharmacol Exp Ther.* 2002 Sep; 302(3):1055–1061.
8. **Rx List Inc.** Denosumab. Available at: www.rxlist.com/ prolia-drug/clinical-pharmacology.htm. Accessed Jan 2016.
9. **Rx List Inc.** Avastin. Available at: www.rxlist.com/avastin-drug. htm. Accessed Jan 2016.
10. **Mena AC, Pulido EG, Guillen-Ponce C.** Understanding the molecular-based mechanism of action of the tyrosine kinase inhibitor: sunitinib. *Anticancer Drugs.* 2010 Jan; 21 (1 Suppl):S3–11.
11. **American Dental Association Council on Scientific Affairs.** Dental management of patients receiving oral bisphosphonate therapy: expert panel recommendations. *J Am Dent Assoc.* 2006 Aug; 137(8):1144–1150.
12. **Marx RE, Sawatari Y, Fortin M, et al.** Bisphosphonate-induced exposed bone (osteonecrosis/osteopetrosis) of the jaws: risk factors, recognition, prevention, and treatment. *J Oral Maxillofac Surg.* 2005 Nov; 63(11):1567–1575.
13. **Lasseter KC, Porras AG, Denker A, et al.** Pharmacokinetic considerations in determining the terminal elimination half-lives of bisphosphonates. *Clin Drug Investig.* 2005; 25(2):107–114.
14. **Marx RE, Cillo JE, Jr.**, Ulloa JJ. Oral bisphosphonate-induced osteonecrosis: risk factors, prediction of risk using serum CTX testing, prevention, and treatment. *J Oral Maxillofac Surg.* 2007 Dec; 65(12):2397–2410.
15. **Marx RE.** *Oral and Intravenous Bisphosphonate-Induced Osteonecrosis of the Jaws. History, Etiology, Prevention, and Treatment.* 2nd Ed. Chicago: Quintessence Pub Co; 2011.
16. **Aghaloo TL, Kang B, Sung EC, et al.** Periodontal disease and bisphosphonates induce osteonecrosis of the jaws in the rat. *J Bone Miner Res.* 2011 Aug; 26(8):1871–1882.
17. **Lenart BA, Lorich DG, Lane JM.** Atypical fractures of the femoral diaphysis in postmenopausal women taking alendronate. *N Engl J Med.* 2008 Mar; 358(12):1304–1306.
18. **Abrahamsen B, Eiken P, Eastell R.** Subtrochanteric and diaphyseal femur fractures in patients treated with alendronate: a register-based national cohort study. *J Bone Miner Res.* 2009 Jun; 24(6):1095–1102.
19. **Neviaser AS, Lane JM, Lenart BA, et al.** Low-energy femoral shaft fractures associated with alendronate use. *J Orthop Trauma.* 2008 May-Jun; 22(5):346–350.

6 Pathogenesis of antiresorptive drug-related osteonecrosis of the jaw

Riham Fliefel, Sven Otto

1 Introductory questions

In this chapter, three questions are raised and discussed:

- Which theories exist for the pathogenesis of antiresorptive drug-related osteonecrosis of the jaw (ARONJ)?
- Why are the jaw bones predominantly affected?
- Why can nitrogen-containing bisphosphonates and denosumab cause ARONJ?

2 Background

Bones are constantly remodeled through osteoblastic (bone formation) and osteoclastic (bone resorption) activity to maintain skeletal strength and integrity. However, imbalance between these phenomena affects bone mineral density leading to such bone disorders as osteoporosis, Paget's disease, myeloma, bone metastases secondary to cancer, as well as osteogenesis imperfecta and inflammatory bone loss. One of the recent treatments of bone disorders is the use of antiresorptive drugs including hormone replacement therapy, selective estrogen receptor modulators, bisphosphonates, and denosumab, which reduce the occurrence of bone pain, pathological fracture, and spinal cord compression [1–4].

Among the antiresorptive drugs, bisphosphonates (BPs) are stable analogues of natural inorganic pyrophosphates [5–7]. They can be classified into nonnitrogen BPs, which metabolically interfere with adenosine triphosphate-dependent (ATP) intracellular pathways, and nitrogen BPs, which inhibit farnesyl pyrophosphate synthase [8, 9]. Denosumab is a new antiresorptive drug with a novel mechanism of action [10]. Both denosumab and bisphosphonates target osteoclasts, however, their effects on osteoblasts are largely indirect [11].

The mechanisms of action of BPs in bone metabolism are complex and multifactorial, altering the osteoclast cytoskeleton, stimulating apoptosis, and reducing proton-pump expression [12–14]. They interfere with chemotaxis and the attachment of osteoclast to bone together with suppressing mature osteoclast function by defective intracellular vesicle transport, which in turn prevents osteoclasts from forming a tight scaling zone or ruffled border required for bone resorption [15–17]. In addition, they inhibit recruitment, activation, and differentiation of osteoclast precursors [18]. The clinical efficacy of BPs rises from their ability to bind strongly to bone mineral [7]. The initial clearance of BPs occurs through renal excretion or adsorption to bone mineral extending over a period of weeks to years [19]. During bone resorption, the acidic pH in the resorption lacuna increases the dissociation of BP from bone [20]. This is followed by the uptake of the BP most likely by fluid-phase endocytosis [21].

Bone resorption is regulated through what is known as RANK/RANKL/OPG pathway [11, 22]. The receptor activator of nuclear factor kappa-B ligand (RANKL) is a transmembrane and soluble protein highly expressed by osteoblasts [23, 24]; its receptor, receptor activator of nuclear factor kappa-B (RANK), is located on the cell membrane of osteoclasts and preosteoclasts [24, 25]. Increased bone resorption results from RANK/RANKL binding, which stimulates the formation, activity, and survival of osteoclasts [26]. Osteoprotegerin (OPG) is a naturally occurring soluble, nonsignaling "decoy receptor" for RANKL. Osteoprotegerin inhibits osteoclast activity by binding to RANKL, preventing its interaction with RANK [26–28]. Both RANKL and OPG are produced by osteoblasts [29].

Denosumab is a fully human monoclonal antibody that was developed specifically to interact with the RANK/RANKL/OPG pathway [7]. By binding to RANKL, it prevents the maturation and differentiation of preosteoclasts in the extracellular environment and promotes apoptosis of osteoclasts [30]. It has several advantages over BPs including better tolerability, ease of subcutaneous injection, shorter half-life, and reduced incidence of nephrotoxicity, rendering it the drug of choice for patients with renal diseases or prostate cancer [31]. In contrast to the BPs, denosumab does not become embedded within bone tissue [10, 11]. Denosumab is cleared from the bloodstream through the reticuloendothelial system, with a half-life of approximately 26 days without inducing the formation of neutralizing antibodies [32].

Antiresorptive drugs have serveral side effects including upper gastrointestinal, where nausea, vomiting, epigastric pain, and dyspepsia can occur after oral administration of drugs for the treatment of osteoporosis. Subsequently, several cases of renal failure were reported following the use of intravenous BPs. A possible mechanism of renal toxicity was the strong affinity of the BP for metal ions and their tendency to form complexes and aggregates with metal ions. Nonspecific conjunctivitis is the most common ocular side effect of BPs, which usually improves without therapy and despite continuing treatment with BPs. Transient hypocalcaemia with secondary hyperparathyroidism is also a side effect of BP administration. There is a possibility of severe and sometimes incapacitating bone, joint, and/or muscle (musculoskeletal) pain in patients taking BPs [33, 34].

3   Theories for the pathogenesis of ARONJ

No potential adverse effect of antiresorptive drugs has caused more scientific attention than ARONJ, which ranges in severity from painless small areas of exposed bone, to significant bone exposure associated with severe pain, sequestration, infection, fistula, or jaw fracture [35–38]. The pathogenesis of the disease is certainly associated with many questions regarding the potential mechanisms underlying the pathophysiology [22, 39, 40]. Five main mechanisms have also been proposed: 1) impaired remodeling; 2) inhibition of angiogenesis; 3) local toxicity; 4) immunomodulation; and 5) infections. It is most likely that a combination of these facilitate the development of ARONJ [41]. However, the most cited theory to explain the mechanism suggests that it is caused by cessation of bone remodeling and bone turnover by the inhibition of osteoclasts [42].

Antiresorptive drug-related osteonecrosis of the jaw most commonly occurs in the oral cavity as the jaws are covered and protected only by a thin layer of periosteum and epithelium against the multitude of bacteria in the oral cavity making it prone for infections. The alveolar bone of the jaws is daily remodeled with a high rate of bone turnover, and the presence of teeth and gum provides an easy entrance

for bacterial infection [40, 43]. The oral structures are subjected to a wide variety of stresses, which may be physiologic, iatrogenic, or inflammatory. The constant stress leads to trauma to the mucosa with exposure of bone [40]. Prolonged use of BPs can suppress bone turnover with accumulation of microcracks resulting in decreased biomechanical competence [35, 44]. Bisphosphonates cause excessive reduction of bone turnover resulting in an increased risk of bone necrosis in osseous repair [45, 46]. However, this theory failed to explain why exposed necrotic lesions are rarely seen in bones other than the jaw. Antiresorptive drug-related osteonecrosis of the jaw does not appear to occur in other conditions associated with reduced bone turnover, such as hypoparathyroidism, and in patients with reported ARONJ the bone turnover markers were not overly suppressed [47, 48]. In patients with breast cancer and bone metastases treated with zoledronate or denosumab, bone scintigraphy images suggest that the bone turnover of the mandible and maxilla is not overly changed when compared to other bones [49].

Blood supply may play a role in ARONJ as its reduction might lead to delayed wound healing due to the antiangiogenic effect [50]. Antiresorptive medications may inhibit angiogenesis by inhibiting the formation of blood vessels, endothelial cells, fibroblast growth factor, and endothelial growth factor impairing endothelial cell (EC) functions leading to altered adhesion and migration. Furthermore, there is reduced proliferation, increased apoptosis, and decreased capillary-like tube formation in ECs that might cause bone necrosis [51–53]. In a study by Wehrhan et al [54], mucoperiosteal tissue samples from ARONJ patients under BPs and controls were assessed for vascularization with CD31 staining and neoangiogenesis by CD105. Although there was no difference in the vascularization between sample groups, there were significantly fewer CD105-positive vessels in ARONJ samples suggesting that neoangiogenesis was suppressed in ARONJ patients. Histological evaluation of ARONJ tissue revealed decreased p63 gene expression, indicating a reduction in basal cell progenitors, and might lead to impaired healing of the oral mucosa [55]. Although BPs, bevacizumab, and sunitinib all have antiangiogenic effects, the effects of denosumab on angiogenesis is largely unknown [56–58]. As such, impaired vascularization may play only a minor role in the development of ARONJ [59].

Soft-tissue cytotoxicity might also play a role explaining why bone is directly exposed to the oral environment through teeth and periodontal ligaments [60]. Local infection and tooth extraction could result in the release of BPs into the local tissues. Provided that the local concentration of drugs is high enough, the proliferation of adjacent epithelial cells could be inhibited and thus slow down the healing of the breached mucosal barrier [61]. However, soft-tissue toxicity has not been reported with denosumab. Use of BPs was explored on a variety of cells, including gastrointestinal cells, cervical epithelial cells, renal cells, prostate epithelial cells, and oral mucosal cells [40]. Antiresorptive drugs also act on immunity, resulting in impairment of myeloid cell function [62, 63], and dendritic cell [64] and T-cell upregulation [65]. They increase the antigenicity of cancer cells as targets and increase adaptive immunity. This impairment of local immunity with an infectious tendency may be a key element in ARONJ [41].

4 Special properties of jaw bones

Infection and periodontal disease are critical factors associated with ARONJ. However, controversy exists as to whether: 1) BP inhibition of bone remodeling results in necrosis with subsequent infection or 2) the direct toxic effects of BPs on the oral mucosa allow for invasion of oral pathogens causing infection with subsequent necrosis [66, 67]. Among all the bones, the jaw seems to be the most liable to bacterial infection since mucosa covering the alveolar bone is very thin and vulnerable and teeth easily become a pathway for bacteria from the outside into the bone. After administration, BPs accumulate in the bone and during physiological remodeling, osteocytes are exposed to BPs in bone [68]. Bisphosphonates bind to bone at neutral pH and are released from bone in an acidic milieu; thus, pH and infections might play an important role in the pathogenesis of ARONJ. This physiologic mechanism takes place in the resorption lacunas during bone resorption, where acid pH increases the dissociation between BP and hydroxyapatite. To date, this well-known feature has usually not been brought into connection to the pathogenesis of ARONJ, but may prove to be the missing part in the multifactorial puzzle [69, 70].

Aghaloo et al [71] found that necrosis of the alveolar bones developed after the placement of a wire ligature around the crown of a maxillary molar in a rat periodontal disease model. The results showed that periodontitis, which is presumably infection-related, can trigger osteonecrosis. When periodontitis occurs, inflammatory cells are recruited to the sites to eliminate the causative pathogens. However, the blockade of bone resorption with BPs may render it difficult for these cells to access the pathogens, allowing the infection to persist. The resulting accumulation of bacterial toxins and inflammation-generated superoxides will promote bone necrosis [68]. The mechanism of ARONJ is highly related to immunity and infection rather than being aseptic or avascular in origin [56]. It mostly follows invasive dental procedures, suggesting that ARONJ likely involves a drug-related compromise in the bone response to invasive trauma. Antiresorptive drug-related osteonecrosis of the jaw often manifests after dental extractions but it has to be taken into consideration that the majority of those extractions are performed due to dental infections, especially apical and periodontal infections. For a direct in vivo mechanism to be identified, it is yet unclear whether invasive trauma by itself is sufficient to precipitate ARONJ in individuals treated with antiresorptive drugs [36, 48]. Polymicrobial infection and periodontal disease are very likely to contribute to the development of ARONJ as a biofilm-associated infection. Filleul et al [72] found out that actinomyces were present in 70% of all cases. Thumbigere-Math et al [73] found actinomyces-like microorganisms in all bone specimens of patients during microbiological examination. In animal models treated with BPs, bacterial infection was sufficient enough to cause ARONJ [36]. Sterile inflammation alone in the soft tissues surrounding the jaw seems insufficient to induce ARONJ [74]. Treatment with antibiotics in animal models [75] and mucoperiosteal coverage on the day of tooth extraction in a rat model prevented the development of ARONJ [76].

The presence of the infectious component in ARONJ seems to be the most dangerous aspect. Oral pathogens should be prevented from reaching the bone surface, and optimum oral hygiene is essential. The current regimens, which consist of oral antiseptics and antibiotics, are not always successful. Ideally, treatment aims to eradicate the underlying infection, prevent secondary infection, stop the disease process, and control symptoms [77]. Traumatic intervention should be avoided, but where it must be undertaken, strict adherence is necessary. The proposed sequence of events in the development of ARONJ with infection could justify temporary discontinuation of the drug to allow recovery of macrophage production and function [78]. A potential scheme for the pathogenesis of ARONJ taking together the above mentioned aspects but stressing the role of local infections is illustrated in **Fig 6-1**. Infection might also be the initiating event for ARONJ in patients receiving denosumab as there is also a strong remodeling suppression and therefore only limited capacity to deal with odontogenic infections.

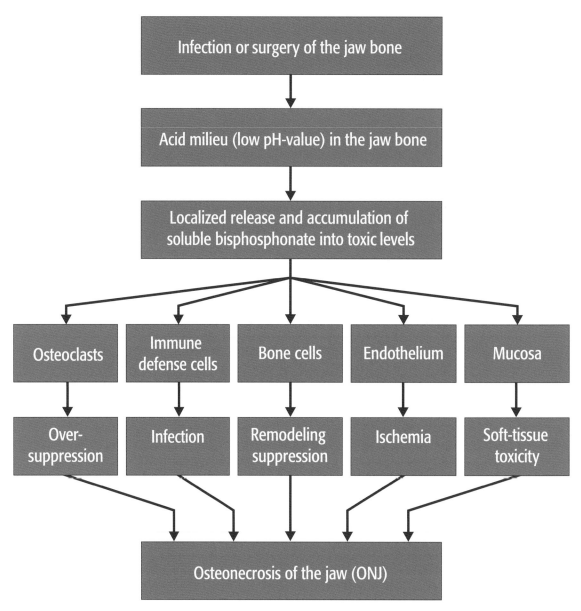

Fig 6-1   Potential scheme for the pathogenesis of ARONJ.

5 Conclusion

While various theories for the etiology of ARONJ are discussed, there is more and more data supporting the important role of local infections. Consequently, the jaw bones, especially in areas with dentoalveolar infections and surgeries, are mainly affected. The similarities and potential differences between ARONJ lesions caused by BPs and denosumab still have to be elucidated.

6 References

1. **Feurer E, Chapurlat R.** Emerging drugs for osteoporosis. *Expert Opin Emerg Drugs.* 2014 Sep; 19(3):385–395.
2. **Boyle WJ, Simonet WS, Lacey DL.** Osteoclast differentiation and activation. *Nature.* 2003 May; 423(6937):337–342.
3. **Russell RG.** Pharmacological diversity among drugs that inhibit bone resorption. *Curr Opin Pharmacol.* 2015 Jun; 22:115–130.
4. **Van den Wyngaert T, Huizing MT, Fossion E, et al.** Bisphosphonates in oncology: rising stars or fallen heroes. *Oncologist.* 2009 Feb; 14(2):181–191.
5. **Fleisch H.** Development of bisphosphonates. *Breast Cancer Res.* 2002; 4(1):30–34.
6. **Russell RG, Watts NB, Ebetino FH, et al.** Mechanisms of action of bisphosphonates: similarities and differences and their potential influence on clinical efficacy. *Osteoporosis International.* 2008 Jun; 19(6):733–759.
7. **Hanley DA, Adachi JD, Bell A, et al.** Denosumab: mechanism of action and clinical outcomes. *Int J Clin Pract.* 2012 Dec; 66(12)1139–1146.
8. **Russell RG.** Bisphosphonates: the first 40 years. *Bone.* 2011 Jul; 49(1):2–19.
9. **Reszka AA, Rodan GA.** Mechanism of action of bisphosphonates. *Curr Osteoporos Rep.* 2003 Sep; 1(2):45–52.
10. **Moen MD, Keam SJ.** Denosumab: a review of its use in the treatment of postmenopausal osteoporosis. *Drugs Aging.* 2011 Jan; 28(1):63–82.
11. **Baron R, Ferrari S, Russell RG.** Denosumab and bisphosphonates: different mechanisms of action and effects. *Bone.* 2011 Apr; 48(4):677–692.
12. **Sato M, Grasser W, Endo N, et al.** Bisphosphonate action. Alendronate localization in rat bone and effects on osteoclast ultrastructure. *J Clin Invest.* 1991 Dec; 88(6):2095–2105.
13. **Hughes DE, Wright KR, Uy HL, et al.** Bisphosphonates promote apoptosis in murine osteoclasts in vitro and in vivo. *J Bone Miner Res.* 1995 Oct; 10(10):1478–1487.
14. **Miller SC, Jee WS.** The effect of dichloromethylene diphosphonate, a pyrophosphate analog, on bone and bone cell structure in the growing rat. *Anat Rec.* 1979 Mar; 193(3):439–462.
15. **Green J.** Cytosolic pH regulation in osteoblasts. *Miner Electrolyte Metab.* 1994; 20(1-2):16–30.
16. **Flanagan AM, TJ Chambers.** Inhibition of bone resorption by bisphosphonates: interactions between bisphosphonates, osteoclasts, and bone. *Calcif Tissue Int.* 1991 Dec; 49(6):407–415.
17. **Coxon FP, Helfrich MH, Van't Hof R, et al.** Protein geranylgeranylation is required for osteoclast formation, function, and survival: inhibition by bisphosphonates and GGTI-298. *J Bone Miner Res.* 2000 Aug; 15(8):1467–1476.
18. **Hughes DE, MacDonald BR, Russell RG, et al.** Inhibition of osteoclast-like cell formation by bisphosphonates in long-term cultures of human bone marrow. *J Clin Invest.* 1989 Jun; 83(6):1930–1935.
19. **Russell RG, Rogers MJ.** Bisphosphonates: from the laboratory to the clinic and back again. *Bone.* 1999 Jul; 25(1):97–106.
20. **Ebetino FH, Francis MD.** Mechanisms of action of etidronate and other bisphosphonates. *Rev Cont Pharmaco.* 1998; 9:233–243.
21. **Thompson K, Rogers MJ, Coxon FP, et al.** Cytosolic entry of bisphosphonate drugs requires acidification of vesicles after fluid-phase endocytosis. *Mol Pharmacol.* 2006 May; 69(5):1624–1632.
22. **Yamashita J, McCauley LK.** Antiresorptives and osteonecrosis of the jaw. *J Evid Based Dent Pract.* 2012 Sep; 12(3 Suppl):S233–247.
23. **Collin-Osdoby P.** Regulation of vascular calcification by osteoclast regulatory factors RANKL and osteoprotegerin. *Circ Res.* 2004 Nov; 95(11):1046–1057.
24. **Lewiecki EM.** Treatment of osteoporosis with denosumab. *Maturitas.* 2010 Jun; 66(2):182–186.
25. **Hsu H, Lacey DL, Dunstan CR, et al.** Tumor necrosis factor receptor family member RANK mediates osteoclast differentiation and activation induced by osteoprotegerin ligand. *Proc Natl Acad Sci USA.* 1999 Mar; 96(7):3540–3545.
26. **Lacey DL, Timms E, Tan HL, et al.** Osteoprotegerin ligand is a cytokine that regulates osteoclast differentiation and activation. *Cell.* 1998 Apr; 93(2):165–176.
27. **Burgess TL, Qian Y, Kaufman S, et al.** The ligand for osteoprotegerin (OPGL) directly activates mature osteoclasts. *J Cell Biol.* 1999 May; 145(3):527–538.
28. **Simonet WS, Lacey DL, Dunstan CR, et al.** Osteoprotegerin: a novel secreted protein involved in the regulation of bone density. *Cell.* 1997 Apr; 89(2):309–319.
29. **Schwarz EM, Ritchlin CT.** Clinical development of anti-RANKL therapy. *Arthritis Res Ther.* 2007; 9(1 Suppl):S7.
30. **Bekker PJ, Holloway D, Nakanishi A, et al.** The effect of a single dose of osteoprotegerin in postmenopausal women. *J Bone Miner Res.* 2001 Feb; 16(2):348–360.
31. **Uyanne J, Calhoun CC, Le AD.** Antiresorptive Drug–Related Osteonecrosis of the Jaw. *Dent Clin North Am.* 2014 Apr; 58(2):369–384.
32. **Amgen Canada Inc.** Prolia product monograph. Canada; Oct 2011.
33. **Kennel KA, Drake MT.** Adverse effects of bisphosphonates: implications for osteoporosis management. *Mayo Clin Proc.* 2009 Jul; 84(7):632–7;quiz 638.

34. **Papapetrou PD.** Bisphosphonate-associated adverse events. *Hormones (Athens).* 2009; 8(2):96–110.

35. **Khosla S, Burr D, Cauley J, et al.** Bisphosphonate-associated osteonecrosis of the jaw: report of a task force of the American Society for Bone and Mineral Research. *J Bone Miner Res.* 2007 Oct; 22(10):1479–1491.

36. **Ruggiero SL, Dodson TB, Fantasia J, et al.** American Association of Oral and Maxillofacial Surgeons position paper on medication-related osteonecrosis of the jaw—2014 update. *J Oral Maxillofac Surg.* 2014 Oct; 72(10):1938–1956.

37. **Lipton A, Fizazi K, Stopeck AT, et al.** Superiority of denosumab to zoledronic acid for prevention of skeletal-related events: a combined analysis of 3 pivotal, randomised, phase 3 trials. *Eur J Cancer.* 2012 Nov; 48(16):3082–3092.

38. **Ruggiero SL, Dodson TB, Assael LA, et al.** American Association of Oral and Maxillofacial Surgeons position paper on bisphosphonate-related osteonecrosis of the jaw—2009 update. *J Oral Maxillofac Surg.* 2009 May; 67(5 Suppl):S2–12.

39. **Allen MR, Burr DB.** The pathogenesis of bisphosphonate-related osteonecrosis of the jaw: so many hypotheses, so few data. *J Oral Maxillofac Surg.* 2009 May; 67(5 Suppl):S61–70.

40. **Landesberg R, Woo V, Cermers S, et al.** Potential pathophysiological mechanisms in osteonecrosis of the jaw. *Ann NY Acad Sci.* 2011 Feb; 1218:62–79.

41. **Wimalawansa SJ.** Insight into bisphosphonate-associated osteomyelitis of the jaw: pathophysiology, mechanisms and clinical management. *Expert Opin Drug Saf.* 2008 Jul; 7(4):491–512.

42. **Marx RE, Sawstari Y, Fortin M, et al.** Bisphosphonate-induced exposed bone (osteonecrosis/osteopetrosis) of the jaws: risk factors, recognition, prevention, and treatment. *J Oral Maxillofac Surg.* 2005 Nov; 63(11):1567–1575.

43. **Yoneda T.** Bisphosphonate-related osteonecrosis of the jaw: position paper from the Allied Task Force Committee of Japanese Society for Bone and Mineral Research, Japan Osteoporosis Society, Japanese Society of Periodontology, Japanese Society for Oral and Maxillofacial Radiology, and Japanese Society of Oral and Maxillofacial Surgeons. *J Bone Miner Metab.* 2010; 28(4):365–383.

44. **Woo SB, Hellstein JW, Kalmar JR.** Narrative [corrected] review: bisphosphonates and osteonecrosis of the jaws. *Ann Intern Med.* 2006; 144(10):753–761.

45. **Chapurlat RD, Arlot M, Burt-Pichat B, et al.** Microcrack frequency and bone remodeling in postmenopausal osteoporotic women on long-term bisphosphonates: a bone biopsy study. *J Bone Miner Res.* 2007 Oct; 22(10):1502–1509.

46. **Stepan JJ, Burr DB, Pavo I, et al.** Low bone mineral density is associated with bone microdamage accumulation in postmenopausal women with osteoporosis. *Bone.* 2007 Sep; 41(3):378–385.

47. **Pazianas M.** Osteonecrosis of the jaw and the role of macrophages. *J Natl Cancer Inst.* 2011 Feb; 103(3):232–240.

48. **Reid IR, Cornish J.** Epidemiology and pathogenesis of osteonecrosis of the jaw. *Nat Rev Rheumatol.* 2012 Nov; 8(2):90–96.

49. **Ristow O, Gerngross C, Schwaiger M, et al.** Effect of antiresorptive drugs on bony turnover in the jaw: denosumab compared with bisphosphonates. *Br J Oral Maxillofac Surg.* 2014 Apr; 52(4):308–313.

50. **Ruggiero SL, Mehrotra B, Rosenberg TJ, et al.** Osteonecrosis of the jaws associated with the use of bisphosphonates: A review of 63 cases. *J Oral Maxillofac Surg.* 2004 May; 62(5):527–534.

51. **Pickett FA.** Bisphosphonate-associated osteonecrosis of the jaw: a literature review and clinical practice guidelines. *J Dent Hyg.* 2006; 80(3):10.

52. **Wood J, Bonjean K, Ruetz S, et al.** Novel antiangiogenic effects of the bisphosphonate compound zoledronic acid. *J Pharmacol Exp Ther.* 2002 Sep; 302(3):1055–1061.

53. **Fournier P, Boissier S, Filleur S, et al.** Bisphosphonates inhibit angiogenesis in vitro and testosterone-stimulated vascular regrowth in the ventral prostate in castrated rats. *Cancer Res.* 2002 Nov 15; 62(22):6538–6544.

54. **Wehrhan F, Stockmann P, Nkenke E, et al.** Differential impairment of vascularization and angiogenesis in bisphosphonate-associated osteonecrosis of the jaw-related mucoperiosteal tissue. *Oral Surg Oral Med Oral Pathol Oral Radiol Endod.* 2011 Aug; 112(2):216–221

55. **Scheller EL, Baldwin CM, Kuo S, et al.** Bisphosphonates inhibit expression of p63 by oral keratinocytes. *J Dent Res.* 2011 Jul; 90(7):894–899.

56. **Roelofs AJ, Thompson K, Gordon S, et al.** Molecular mechanisms of action of bisphosphonates: current status. *Clin Cancer Res.* 2006 Oct 15; 12(20 Pt 2):6222s–6230s.

57. **Koch FP, Walter C, Hansen T, et al.** Osteonecrosis of the jaw related to sunitinib. *Oral Maxillofac Surg.* 2011 Mar; 15(1):63–66.

58. **Misso G, Porru M, Stoppacciaro M, et al.** Evaluation of the in vitro and in vivo antiangiogenic effects of denosumab and zoledronic acid. *Cancer Biol Ther.* 2012 Dec; 13(14):1491–1500.

59. **Compston J.** Pathophysiology of atypical femoral fractures and osteonecrosis of the jaw. *Osteoporos Int.* 2011 Dec; 22(12):2951–2961.

60. **Badel T, Pavicin IS, Carek AJ, et al.** Pathophysiology of osteonecrosis of the jaw in patients treated with bisphosphonate. *Coll Antropol.* 2013 Jun; 37(2):645–651.

61. **Cornish J, Bava U, Callon KE, et al.** Bone-bound bisphosphonate inhibits growth of adjacent non-bone cells. *Bone.* 2011 Oct; 49(4):710–716

62. **Melani C, Sangaletti S, Barazzetta FM, et al.** Amino-biphosphonate-mediated MMP-9 inhibition breaks the tumor-bone marrow axis responsible for myeloid-derived suppressor cell expansion and macrophage infiltration in tumor stroma. *Cancer Res.* 2007 Dec; 67(23):11438–11446.

63. **Dieli F, Vermijlen D, Fulfaro F, et al.** Targeting human {gamma delta} T cells with zoledronate and interleukin-2 for immunotherapy of hormone-refractory prostate cancer. *Cancer Res.* 2007 Aug; 67(15):7450–7457.

64. **Fiore F, Castella B, Nuschak B, et al.** Enhanced ability of dendritic cells to stimulate innate and adaptive immunity on short-term incubation with zoledronic acid. *Blood.* 2007 Aug; 110(3):921–927.

65. **Sato K, Kimura S, Segawa H, et al.** Cytotoxic effects of gammadelta T cells expanded ex vivo by a third generation bisphosphonate for cancer immunotherapy. *Int J Cancer.* 2005 Aug 10; 116(1):94–99.

66. **Roodman GD.** Mechanisms of bone metastasis, pathophysiology of osteonecrosis of the jaw, and integrins, platelets and bone metastasis: meeting report from skeletal complications of malignancy V. *IBMS BoneKEy.* 2008; 5(8):294–296.

67. **Anavi-Lev K, Anavi Y, Chaushu G, et al.** Bisphosphonate related osteonecrosis of the jaws: clinico-pathological investigation and histomorphometric analysis. *Oral Surg Oral Med Oral Pathol Oral Radiol.* 2013 May; 115(5):660–6

68. **Ikebe T.** Pathophysiology of BRONJ: Drug-related osteoclastic disease of the jaw. *Oral Science Internatl.* 2013; 10(1):1–8.

69. **Otto S, Pautke C, Opelz C, et al.** Osteonecrosis of the Jaw: Effect of Bisphosphonate Type, Local Concentration, and Acidic Milieu on the Pathomechanism. *J Oral Maxillofac Surg.* 2010 Nov; 68(11):2837–2845

70. **Otto S, Hafner S, Mast G, et al.** Bisphosphonate-related osteonecrosis of the jaw: is pH the missing part in the pathogenesis puzzle? *J Oral Maxillofac Surg.* 2010 May; 68(5):1158–1161.

71. **Aghaloo TL, Kang B, Sung EC, et al.** Periodontal disease and bisphosphonates induce osteonecrosis of the jaws in the rat. *J Bone Miner Res.* 2011 Aug; 26(8):1871–1882.

72. **Filleul O, Crompot E, Saussez S.** Bisphosphonate-induced osteonecrosis of the jaw: a review of 2,400 patient cases. *J Cancer Res Clin Oncol.* 2010 Aug; 136(8):1117–1124.

73. **Thumbigere-Math V, Sabino MC, Gopalakrishnan R, et al.** Bisphosphonate-Related Osteonecrosis of the Jaw: Clinical Features, Risk Factors, Management, and Treatment Outcomes of 26 Patients. *J Oral Maxillofac Surg.* 2009 Sep; 67(9):1904–1913.

74. **Bonnet N, Lesclous P, Saffar JL, et al.** Zoledronate effects on systemic and jaw osteopenias in ovariectomized periostin-deficient mice. *PLoS One.* 2013; 8(3):e58726.

75. **López-Jornet P, Camacho-Alonso F, Martínez-Canovas A, et al.** Perioperative antibiotic regimen in rats treated with pamidronate plus dexamethasone and subjected to dental extraction: a study of the changes in the jaws. *J Oral Maxillofac Surg.* 2011 Oct; 69(10):2488–2493.

76. **Abtahi J, Agholme F, Aspenberg P.** Prevention of osteonecrosis of the jaw by mucoperiosteal coverage in a rat model. *Int J Oral Maxillofac Surg.* 2013 May; 42(5):632–636.

77. **McLeod NM, Patel V, Kusanale A, et al.** Bisphosphonate osteonecrosis of the jaw: a literature review of UK policies versus international policies on the management of bisphosphonate osteonecrosis of the jaw. *Br J Oral Maxillofac Surg.* 2011 Jul; 49(5):335–342.

78. **Katsarelis H, Shah NP, Dhariwal DK, et al.** Infection and medication-related osteonecrosis of the jaw. *J Dent Res.* 2015 Apr; 94(4):534–539.

7 Small animal models for antiresorptive drug-related osteonecrosis of the jaw

James L Borke, Ezher H Dayisoylu, Stephan Zeiter

1 Introductory questions

In this chapter, the following questions are raised and discussed:

- Does small animal investigation make sense?
- What are the opportunities and limitations of small animal investigation?
- What are the advantages and disadvantages of small animal models of antiresorptive drug-related osteonecrosis of the jaw (ARONJ)?
- What controversies exist concerning these small animal models?
- Are there significant differences among the various small animal models of ARONJ?
- Does jaw size matter?

2 The role of small animal investigation

The role of animal models in scientific investigation is well established, however, with regard to size, the specific line of investigation needs to be taken into account. The genomic sequences for mice and rats have been available for several years. Both species are now known to share about 98% of their genes with humans [1, 2]. In mice for example, of the 4000 or so genes that have been studied, only about 10 have been found in mice or humans and not the other species [3]. This, however, does not tell the whole story. The mouse Encyclopedia of DNA Elements (ENCODE) project has been creating a comprehensive catalog of functional elements in the mouse genome, and is comparing these elements to those in the human genome [4]. These elements include the genes that code for proteins, but also nonprotein-coding genes, and regulatory segments that control the turning on and off of genes. These regions are not as well conserved and need to be closely monitored in studies comparing specific regulatory differences.

In addition to genetic and molecular differences, differences between the structure of animal and human tissues must also be considered. A study by Bagi et al in 2011 compared bone anatomy in commonly used laboratory animal models with humans [5]. They found that in rabbits and rodents, the small amounts of cancellous bone as well as the lack of Haversian canals in the mandible limited the use of these animals as preclinical models for dental research. However, in the same study, the authors suggest that rodent models, particularly rats, are often very useful models for conducting basic research involving the skeleton when differences in species are considered. The many recent publications in ARONJ research support the use of rats for this purpose.

When using a small animal as a model for ARONJ, molecular and tissue differences may be less important than mechanical and metabolic considerations. For example, differences in bite force, the effect of diet on the oral microbiota, as well as the higher rate of metabolism found in rodents all contribute to the time course and effects of drug distribution uptake and utilization impacting the development of ARONJ.

The long answer to the question of whether small animal investigation makes sense for the study of the development, mechanisms, and treatment of ARONJ, therefore requires a careful analysis of the parameters being investigated in each individual study and the impact of species differences on the results.

3 Opportunities and limitations of small animal investigations

The decision to use small animal models as research subjects involves factors of both a nonscientific and a scientific nature. The lower cost for acquiring and housing small animals rather than large animals is often a major factor in the decision to use small animals as models. Studies involving human research subjects are also not ideal as these involve additional regulations necessary to protect human research subjects. However, from a scientific point of view, animals often make better research subjects than human beings. The differences between individual human subjects in lifestyle, diet, and genetics, even for age and gender-matched individuals from the same community, introduce additional variables that cannot be controlled for in human studies. Another major advantage to using small animals as research subjects is that laboratory mice and rats have a much shorter life cycle. Because rats and mice live for only two to three years, researchers can study the effects of treatments or genetic manipulation over an entire lifespan, or across multiple generations. Studies of this type are generally not feasible using human subjects or large animals.

Conversely, as mentioned in the previous section, there are disadvantages to using small animals as models for some disorders. In ARONJ for example, the short ~2-year life span of a rat may not allow enough time for development of the disorder with exposure to a drug at a dose that is equivalent to the human dose, which could require up to 10 years to manifest. Small animals may require additional interventions or higher levels of bisphosphonates (BPs) or other necrosis-inducing agents to manifest ARONJ over their short life. However, several studies to date have demonstrated that it is very possible to produce ARONJ in the rat model [7] (and see Howie et al [6] for a review of recent models)

(**Fig 7-1**). The naturally higher metabolic rate of the rat along with surgical trauma, corticosteroids, periodontal disease, or higher dosing conditions have all been exploited to produce small animal ARONJ models with many of the characteristics of human ARONJ (**Fig 7-2**) [8].

The use of small animals as models for ARONJ has recently been advanced by a 2014 publication by de Barros Silva et al [9]. In their study, the authors provide a better calculation of equivalent human dosing for BPs and other drugs used in research involving small animal models. Most published studies involving human-equivalent dosing of small animals calculate the dosage based on mg drug/kg body weight. Based on this method, a 4 mg dose of BP for a 66 kg person would be 0.06 mg/kg, which translates into a 12 µg equivalent dose for a 200 g rat. The de Barros Silva study, however, used the Dose Calculator, Conversion Chemotherapy of Humans to Animals, provided free by the United States Food and Drug Administration [10]. This calculator not only takes into account body weight but also surface area for the pharmacological conversion of the human dose to the dose equivalent for animals. By this method, a dose of 4 mg used to treat multiple myeloma in humans was calculated to be 0.60 mg/kg or an equivalent dose of 120 µg for a 200 g rat, a value 10 times the dose calculated by the earlier method.

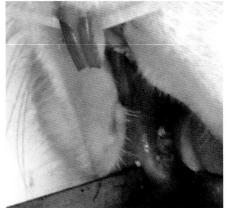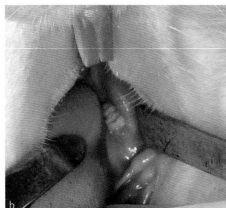

Fig 7-1a–b Extraction sites after 4 weeks [7].
a   Zoledronic acid-treated rat showing nonhealing at the extraction site.
b   Control rat showing a healed extraction site.

(Images with kind permission from the Journal of Oral Implantology, Allen Press Publishing Services).

James L Borke, Ezher II Dayisoylu, Stephan Zeiter

4   Advantages and disadvantages of using small animal models of ARONJ

One of the key advantages of using small animal models involves the medical advances directly attributable to animal research. In 2011, the journal Nature conducted a survey of approximately 1,000 scientists working in the biomedical field. From this survey, greater than 90% of the scientists that responded found the use of animals in research was essential for progress in medical diagnosis and treatment [11]. This collective opinion arises out of the historic contributions of animal research to major medical advancements for well over a century. Some of the advances attributable to research involving animals include the use of rodent models in the development of diagnostic and treatment methods for brain disorders including schizophrenia, Huntington's disease, Alzheimer's, and Parkinson's disease [12]. Other advances include the understanding and treatment of breast cancer, tuberculosis, multiple sclerosis, and childhood leukemia [12]. The pathological processes involved in ARONJ involve multiple tissues including bone, the oral mucosa, and the vasculature. It is therefore reasonable to assume that major future advances in the diagnosis, treatment, and prevention of ARONJ will also arise as a result of studies in living animals containing the multiple cell and tissue types involved and functioning in their natural relationships.

On the negative side of the debate concerning the use of small animal models for ARONJ research are the differences between small animals and humans in their life span, anatomy, metabolism, diets, as well as issues of scale. There are multiple examples in the literature of specific drugs and treatments that were successfully used in animal studies that failed during human trials. This is particularly true for cancer research. An article in the American Journal of Translational Research from 2014 states that the average rate of successful translation from animal models to clinical cancer trials is less than 8% [13]. They report that the vast majority of agents that are found to be successful in animal models are not successful in human trials. While this may, in part, be a function of the unique nature of individual cancers, examples of animal model failures can be seen in most other areas of translational animal investigation as well. An infamous example of this is seen in the trial in London of the drug TGN1412, which was designed as a treatment for rheumatoid arthritis, multiple sclerosis, and certain cancers [14]. This drug was first successfully tested in several animal species at several hundred times the dose given to humans in the trial with no ill effects. However, TGN1412 then caused a catastrophic systemic organ failure in the human subjects injected with only a small amount of the drug. Another example is the use of matrix metalloproteinase (MMP) inhibitors as therapies against arthritis.

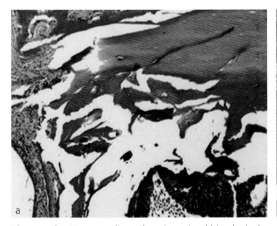
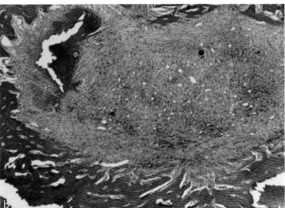

Fig 7-2a–b   Hematoxylin and eosin stained histological sections of mandibular extraction sites 4 weeks after extraction [8].
a   Zoledronic acid-treated rat showing necrotic bone and inflammatory cell infiltrates.
b   Control rat showing normal healing of the extraction site.

(Images with kind permission from the Journal of Cranio-Maxillo-Facial Surgery, Elsevier).

After multiple successful studies in rodents and unsuccessful human trials, only the drug periostat (doxycycline hyclate), a nonspecific MMP inhibitor, has actually been approved for clinical use [15].

With these historic advantages and disadvantages as a background, the careful and measured use of small animal models in ARONJ research would still seem to be the model of choice, depending on the type of research question.

5   Controversies concerning small animal models of ARONJ

Although there are many studies regarding the effect of antiresorptive agents (AR) and the development of osteonecrosis of the jaws, controversy still continues about the use of animal models. The main controversial topics can be listed as follows: age and sex of the animals; application route; dosage and duration of AR; and concomitant interventions. Several authors have noted ARONJ-like lesions with a variety of protocols, but the reproducibility of these lesions are uncertain. Some authors attempted to achieve ARONJ-like lesions via single administration of AR with or without adjuvant agents and noted different rates of necrosis development. On the other hand, repeated systemically administered AR has also been investigated. These too produced various rates of necrosis. Explanations of these differences have been attributed to the surgical interventions, however, it should be noted that the total administered drug dosage is also likely to have been a crucial element.

Jaw bones are reported to have a unique structure that undergoes a high intracortical remodeling rate of approximately 20 times the rate of remodeling of the iliac crest [16]. For this reason, dogs and primates are thought to be good animal models for ARONJ because of their capacity for intracortical bone remodeling. Unfortunately, ethical issues and the high expenses associated with large animal models such as dogs and primates restrict the use of these animals. To mitigate this problem, several attempts were made to stimulate intracortical bone remodeling in rodents by using ovariectomy, but the results were unpredictable [6, 17–19]. Recently, Kim et al tried to achieve a reproducible ARONJ model with ovariectomy but their study produced rats where only 77.8% exhibited ARONJ in the ovariectomized group versus 47.2% exhibiting ARONJ in the simulated surgery group [20].

Injection route is another concern for animal studies. Several investigators have studied ARONJ with subcutaneous, intraperitoneal, intravenous, and also with oral administration routes for drug delivery [6, 21–23]. The outcome of these studies suggests that the intraperitoneal and intravenous routes are the most reliable [6, 23]. In addition to administration method, dosage and duration of exposure to the drugs are also important issues. High doses of AR can lead to systemic toxicity that will undermine the reliability of the studies. Therefore, the dosages should be tested for systemic toxicity by examining the histopathology of tissues such as the kidney and liver. Wounding, steroid injection, vitamin D deficiency, and other chemotherapeutic agents were also tested as concomitant aids in the production of ARONJ models. These modalities, however, were not widely accepted. The exception, however, is tooth extraction. Recent studies clearly show that tooth extraction is a triggering event for the development of ARONJ-like lesions in small animal models [6].

6   Differences between small animal models of ARONJ

There are several studies regarding the development of ARONJ-like lesions in animal models. It should be kept in mind that an animal model should be genetically similar to humans in order to mimic the initiation and progression of the disease. As mentioned in a previous section, mice and rats have now had their genomes mapped. The genetic similarity of rats and mice to humans are both above 95% [24].

Rice rats were one of the earliest animal models for the evaluation of the effects of antiresorptive agents. Gothcher et al used periodontal ligating for a periodontal bone loss model and noted reduced vascular space and increased fibrosis following AR administration [25]. Although the authors did not intend to investigate ARONJ, their result was one of the earliest signs that oral manipulation could lead to bone necrosis. A study by Sonis et al is considered a hallmark for the use of small animal models of ARONJ and clearly showed that trauma is an essential trigger event for the development of ARONJ-like lesions in rats [21]. Sonis et al used 3-month-old rats with three subcutaneous zoledronic acid injections at a dose of 7.5 µg/kg along with 1 mg/kg dexamethasone (DX) at 7,14, or 21 days. The authors also performed tooth extractions following drug administration. Despite the importance of this study, the drug dosage and necrosis rates were considered controversial in their study. Senel et al proposed a different dosage of three injections of ZA in one week of 0.1 mg/kg for 6 weeks without any surgical intervention or concomitant drug administration and found only inflammatory changes [26]. Later, this study group tried the same dosage with surgical intervention and achieved 66% ARONJ and noted tooth extraction is an essential step for ARONJ development in rats [27]. Finally, Howie et al reported using a protocol including repeated trauma to produce ARONJ-like lesions in rats [6]. In this study, the authors used retired-breeder female Spraque-Dawley rats for intravenous ZA injection at a dose of 80 µg/kg for 13 weeks. In this model, tooth extraction was repeated at 13 and 14 weeks. This protocol produced 100% ARONJ-like lesions in this model. In this same study, the authors also investigated the systemic toxicity of the drug. Their results revealed no systemic toxicity at that dosage. Both of these results suggest that their protocol is a reliable model for ARONJ induction. The Howie et al study also reviewed the various studies using rats as models for ARONJ. Together, these studies support the widely accepted view that small animal models are useful and effective tools for ARONJ research as long as careful consideration is given to the age, dosage, and surgical interventions employed.

7   Consideration of scale when using animals

Although rodents are widely studied models for ARONJ development, the small jaw size may influence optimal study design. The smaller jaw size, small oral cavity, as well as smaller tooth size and reduced bite forces can impact the results and limit the translational benefits to humans. For example, tooth extraction of such small teeth in the oral cavity of a rodent is challenging. It is therefore important that tooth extraction be performed by experienced researchers to avoid fracturing of the root tips or excessive trauma leading to inaccurate evaluation of the healing socket. In addition, one of the clinical definitions of ARONJ requires unhealed exposed bone with mucosal ulceration. Such identification can be underestimated on gross examination of such a small area of tissue, especially when only a single tooth is extracted, which in this way can also impact the results. Research would benefit from the standardization of a small animal model of ARONJ based on criteria established and agreed upon by researchers, clinicians, and pathologists working in this area.

8   Conclusion

The discussion in this chapter supports the vital role that small animal models play in the advancement of our knowledge of ARONJ. Understanding of the strengths and limitations of these model systems, however, is an essential requirement for the interpretation of study results as we move forward toward new treatments that circumvent the devastating clinical manifestations of ARONJ.

9   References

1. **Gibbs RA, Weinstock GM, Metzker ML, et al.** Genome sequence of the Brown Norway rat yields insights into mammalian evolution. *Nature.* 2004 Apr; 428(6982):493–521.
2. **Waterston RH, Lindblad-Toh K, Birney E, et al.** Initial sequencing and comparative analysis of the mouse genome. *Nature.* 2002 Dec; 420(6915):520–562.
3. **Yue F, Cheng Y, Breschi A, et al.** A comparative encyclopedia of DNA elements in the mouse genome. *Nature.* 2014 Nov; 515(7527):355–364.
4. **Stamatoyannopoulos JA, Snyder M, Hardison R, et al.** An encyclopedia of mouse DNA elements (Mouse ENCODE). *Genome Biol.* 2012; 13(8):418.
5. **Bagi CM, Berryman E, Moalli MR.** Comparative bone anatomy of commonly used laboratory animals: implications for drug discovery. *Comp Med.* 2011 Feb; 61(1):76–85.
6. **Howie RN, Borke JL, Kurago Z, et al.** A model for osteonecrosis of the jaw with zoledronate treatment following repeated major trauma. *PLoS One.* 2015; 10(7):e0132520. Epub 07/18/2015.
7. **Marino KL, Zakhary I, Abdelsayed RA, et al.** Development of a rat model of bisphosphonate-related osteonecrosis of the jaw (BRONJ). *J Oral Implantol.* 2012 Sep; 38 Spec No:511–518.
8. **Borke JL, McAllister B, Harris T, et al.** Correlation of changes in the mandible and retina/choroid vasculature of a rat model of BRONJ. *J Craniomaxillofac Surg.* 2015 Sep; 43(7):1144–1150.
9. **Silva PG, Ferreira Junior AE, Teofilo CR, et al.** Effect of different doses of zoledronic acid in establishing of bisphosphonate-related osteonecrosis. *Arch Oral Biol.* 2015 Sep; 60(9):1237–1245.
10. **US Food and Drug Administration.** Dose Calculator, Conversion Chemotherapy of Humans to Animals. Available at: www.accessdata.fda.gov. Accessed June 2015.
11. **Cressey D.** Animal research: Battle scars. *Nature.* 2011 Feb 24; 470(7335):452–453.
12. **Quimby F.** Animal models in biomedical research. In: Fox JG, Cohen BJ, Loew F (eds). *Laboratory Animal Medicine.* New York: Academy Press; 2002:1185–1219.
13. **Mak IW, Evaniew N, Ghert M.** Lost in translation: animal models and clinical trials in cancer treatment. *Am J Transl Res.* 2014; 6(2):114–118.
14. **Tabares P, Berr S, Romer PS, et al.** Human regulatory T cells are selectively activated by low-dose application of the CD28 superagonist TGN1412/TAB08. *Eur J Immunol.* 2014 Apr; 44(4):1225–1236.
15. **Pulkoski-Gross AE.** Historical perspective of matrix metalloproteases. *Front Biosci (Schol Ed).* 2015; 7:125–149.
16. **Garetto LP, Chen J, Parr JA, et al.** Remodeling dynamics of bone supporting rigidly fixed titanium implants: a histomorphometric comparison in four species including humans. *Implant Dent.* 1995 Winter; 4(4):235–243. Epub 01/01/1995.
17. **Li CL, Liu XL, Cai WX, et al.** Effect of ovariectomy on stimulating intracortical remodeling in rats. *Biomed Res Int.* 2014; 2014:421431. Epub 10/06/2014.
18. **Kubek DJ, Burr DB, Allen MR.** Ovariectomy stimulates and bisphosphonates inhibit intracortical remodeling in the mouse mandible. *Orthod Craniofac Res.* 2010 Nov; 13(4):214–222. Epub 11/03/2010.
19. **Li CL, Lu WW, Seneviratne CJ, et al.** Role of periodontal disease in bisphosphonate-related osteonecrosis of the jaws in ovariectomized rats. *Clin Oral Implants Res.* 2016 Jan; 27(1):1–6. Epub 11/06/2014.
20. **Kim JW, Tatad JC, Landayan ME, et al.** Animal model for medication-related osteonecrosis of the jaw with precedent metabolic bone disease. *Bone.* 2015 Dec; 81:442–448. Epub 08/25/2015.
21. **Sonis ST, Watkins BA, Lyng GD, et al.** Bony changes in the jaws of rats treated with zoledronic acid and dexamethasone before dental extractions mimic bisphosphonate-related osteonecrosis in cancer patients. *Oral Oncol.* 2009 Feb; 45(2):164–172. Epub 08/22/2008.
22. **Abtahi J, Agholme F, Sandberg O, et al.** Bisphosphonate-induced osteonecrosis of the jaw in a rat model arises first after the bone has become exposed. No primary necrosis in unexposed bone. *J Oral Pathol Med.* 2012 Jul; 41(6):494–499. Epub 01/25/2012.
23. **Dayisoylu EH, Senel FC, Ungor C, et al.** The effects of adjunctive parathyroid hormone injection on bisphosphonate-related osteonecrosis of the jaws: an animal study. *Int J Oral Maxillofac Surg.* 2013 Nov; 42(11):1475–1480. Epub 06/12/2013.
24. **Nilsson S, Helou K, Walentinsson A, et al.** Rat-mouse and rat-human comparative maps based on gene homology and high-resolution zoo-FISH. *Genomics.* 2001 Jun 15; 74(3):287–298. Epub 06/21/2001.
25. **Gotcher JE, Jee WS.** The progress of the periodontal syndrome in the rice rat. I. Morphometric and autoradiographic studies. *J Periodontal Res.* 1981 May; 16(3):275–291. Epub 05/01/1981.
26. **Senel FC, Kadioglu Duman M, Muci E, et al.** Jaw bone changes in rats after treatment with zoledronate and pamidronate. *Oral Surg Oral Med Oral Pathol Oral Radiol Endod.* 2010 Mar; 109(3):385–391. Epub 01/12/2010.
27. **Dayisoylu EH, Ungor C, Tosun E, et al.** Does an alkaline environment prevent the development of bisphosphonate-related osteonecrosis of the jaw? An experimental study in rats. *Oral Surg Oral Med Oral Pathol Oral Radiol.* 2014 Mar; 117(3):329–334. Epub 12/26/2013.

8 Large animal models for antiresorptive drug-related osteonecrosis of the jaw

Matthew R Allen, Pit Voss, Christoph Pautke

1 Introductory questions

In this final chapter, three questions are raised and discussed:
- Can antiresorptive drug-related osteonecrosis of the jaw (ARONJ) be related in large animals?
- Are animal models really necessary?
- What are the advantages of using large animals versus rodents?

2 Introduction

Preclinical studies play an essential role in scientific advancement. Although small animals, such as mice and rats, are the most commonly used preclinical model, there is an important role for large animal models [1]. In most scenarios, results from rodent studies often need to be reproduced in a larger animal model for the findings to advance along the research pipeline. All preclinical model systems have strengths and weaknesses, and in most instances, no one model works best. Although the majority of work in ARONJ has been undertaken using rodents, important studies and advancements have also been made utilizing large animal models [2].

3 Advantages and disadvantages of large animal models

Large animal models, including rabbits, dogs, pigs, sheep, and nonhuman primates, have several important strengths as an animal model for skeletal biology in general, and ARONJ specifically. Anatomically, the jaw and teeth of several large animals closely resemble those of humans. This is in contrast to rodents, which have several sets of molars along with continuously erupting incisions [3]. There is a practical advantage of large animals when it comes to surgical manipulation associated with ARONJ studies. The larger structure that accompanies a large animal makes dental extraction somewhat easier, and more traditional, compared

to smaller animals. The oral microflora of large animals has also been shown to more closely mimic human microflora compared to rodents [4–6].

In humans, dynamic bone cell activity occurs within four different envelopes: periosteal, endocortical, trabecular, and intracortical. Rodents (both mice and rats) undergo activity on the first three, but lack intracortical remodeling. Larger animals, rabbits, pig, sheep, dogs, and nonhuman primates all experience intracortical remodeling. Intracortical remodeling results in larger animals having a distinctly different bone structure at the micro and nanostructure levels compared with rodents. The presence of osteons (Haversian systems) provides regional heterogeneity in mineral, collagen, and water in large animals as exists in humans.

A less appreciated difference between small and large animals in research that has particular implications for ARONJ is the difference in pharmacological dosing. The metabolic rate of rodents is considerably higher than in larger animals (and humans) and thus the pharmacokinetics of drugs is certainly different. This makes it challenging to determine the "clinically-relevant" dose of a drug among species and often makes it difficult to know the role of dose on a particular outcome. For orally delivered drugs, gavage is needed in smaller animals (which can produce significant stress and the associated physiological changes) while in larger animals, traditional oral dosing via tablet/oral suspension is possible.

Although there are several advantages in large animal modeling for skeletal biology research, some disadvantages also exist. Larger animals require a level of housing that may not be possible at all institutions, and there are associated costs that can be prohibitive for large scale studies. Related to this, experiment duration is often lengthened due to the slower rate of the remodeling cycle in large animals (ranging from 2–6 months) as compared with rodents (typically < 1 month). Thus, while it may be possible to study several combinations of treatment/timeframes in a rodent study, it is often necessary to limit group numbers, group sizes, or study duration in large animal studies. The care and use regulations that oversee animal usage are much more extensive for larger animals as compared with rodents, and there is also a difference in public perception regarding the treatment of larger animals involved in research. Finally, a large body of work does not exist, nor is there the same level of research tools (genetic manipulation) for large animals, although the advancement of clustered regularly-interspaced short palindromic repeats (CRISPR) technology may solve the latter.

4   The use of large animals in ARONJ research

4.1   Göttingen minipigs

The Göttingen minipig model was established in 2012. The minipigs (2-year-olds, average weight 38 kg) received weekly zoledronate (ZOL) infusions (2 mg in saline solution, equivalent to 0.05 mg ZOL/kg body weight, comparable to the human dose, although on a more aggressive dosing schedule). Tooth extraction (6 teeth in each animal) was performed after six ZOL administrations, and ZOL infusions were continued for 10 weeks. The jaw bones were harvested and analyzed with computed tomography and histology. Each animal that received ZOL developed the typical signs of jaw bone necrosis with exposed bone in at least

three of the six tooth extraction sites (**Fig 8-1**), while in the control group, no bone exposure was found. Radiologically, the alveolar defects were not replaced by cancellous bone formation in 27 of the 30 extraction sites, and cortical consolidation was observed in only 19 of 30 sites. Typical histopathological signs of bone necrosis (nonvital bone, with rough margins and empty lacunae, no osteocytes) were detected in all but one extraction site (29/30). This study illustrated that jaw bone necrosis could be induced in the minipig model using bisphosphonates (BPs) [4].

In a second study with minipigs, osteonecrosis could be reliably induced. Furthermore, a dose dependency was observed with more severe ARONJ stages under higher ZOL dosages (unpublished results). Under higher BP dosages, ARONJ occurred more frequently in areas with no tooth extractions but with chronic infections.

Göttingen minipigs have a nonseasonal oestrus cycle, a characteristic decrease in bone mineral density following estrogen deficiency, and bone turnover parameters that all similarly exist in humans. With a skeletal biology that closely mimics humans, the finding of jaw bone necrosis with BP treatment makes this a promising candidate that will allow the interplay of drugs and bone turnover to be modeled and analyzed [4].

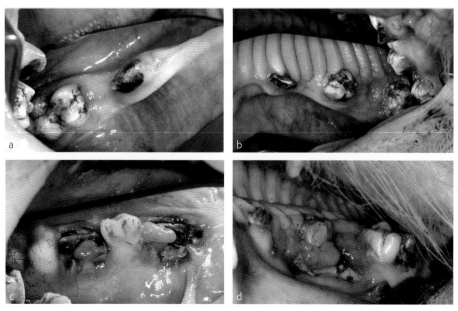

Fig 8-1a–d Intraoral views of a minipig 10 weeks after tooth extractions. Uneventful wound healing occurred in the control group: mandible (**a**) and maxilla (**b**). In contrast, animals in the bisphosphonate group showed impaired healing and exposed bone: mandible (**c**) and maxilla (**d**) [4].

(Images with kind permission from Bone journal, Elsevier).

4.2 Sheep

Sheep are docile and easy to house, and they have cortical and trabecular remodeling cycles and other conditions that are comparable to the human, such as body size, weight, and bone remodeling rates. In establishing a sheep model, 0.075 mg ZOL/kg body weight was infused every third week for 15 weeks before and after extraction of two lower premolars (**Fig 8-2**). All four animals in the study groups developed ARONJ in all extraction sites and the additional periodontal regions of exposed bone, whereas the animals of the control group had uneventful wound healing. These findings were confirmed with μCT, zero echo time MRI, and histology. Interestingly, in sheep treated with ZOL, massive periosteal thickening arose around the extraction sites [7, 8].

The same protocol was conducted in a group of sheep after osteopenia induction using an established protocol with ovariectomy, low calcium diet, and intramuscular administration of glucocorticoids. Unfortunately, two of the animals in the study group were lost before the operative procedure due to poor general health conditions. The remaining animals developed exposed bone at all extraction and several other sites, while the animals of the control group had uneventful wound healing with complete mucosal closure and new bone formation of the extraction sockets. Because of one accidental dose of ZOL during the tooth extraction procedure,

one animal in the control group had to be excluded. Nevertheless, even though this ewe had complete wound closure at the extraction site, it spontaneously developed other regions of exposed bone and a large sequestrum with abnormal tooth mobility.

Being an established model for oral implantology, bone augmentation procedures, and fracture healing, the sheep model encourages new studies in these fields enabling evaluation of the influence of ZOL [7, 8].

4.3 Dogs

The emergence of ONJ (as it was called at the time) in 2003/2004 coincided with a research study in which beagles were being treated for up to 3 years with oral doses of BPs. The initial investigative approach was built on work from the 1960s in which matrix necrosis (that is, loss of osteocyte viability and canaliculi patency) could be assessed with basic fuchsin staining. Portions of the mandibles from vehicle and BP treated animals (alendronate, both at a clinical dose and a 5x clinical dose) were isolated and stained with fuchsin. Following processing of the tissue down to microscopic slides, the tissues were examined for signs of necrosis. While there was no sign of any necrotic regions in the vehicle treated animals, a significant number of the BP treated animals had focal regions of nonviable bone. These ranged in size and

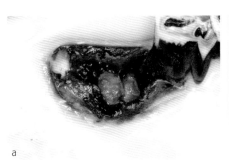
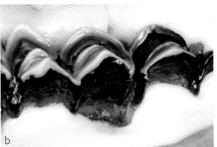

a

b

Fig 8-2a–b An ARONJ lesion with purulent drainage after the extraction of two lower premolars in a sheep (**a**). Spontaneous open bone in the maxilla of the same sheep (**b**).

location, and were not present in all animals (although a comprehensive evaluation of the entire mandible was not undertaken). These results occurred in the setting of significant remodeling suppression, as BP treated dogs had intracortical remodeling rates that were 75% lower than controls. Based on these findings, the working hypothesis emerged that intracortical remodeling suppression in BP animals was leading to the accumulation of nonviable bone and, if additional insult was imparted on a nearby area, that this could start the sequelae of events that culminate in overt ARONJ [9, 10].

Follow-up studies were designed to explore the utility of the dog as a model for ARONJ. In short-term (3 month) studies, overt exposed bone was noted in one BP treated animal following dental extraction. The site eventually formed a sequestrum and then healed. Under the assumption that longer term exposure to BPs, or the combination of BPs and dexamethasone (as was successfully recapitulating ARONJ in rodents at the time) would expand the ability to produce exposed bone, a study was designed in which animals were treated for 9 months prior to dental extractions. There were no cases of exposed bone in this study although there were a number of treated animals that failed to properly heal at the extraction sites, based on CT assessment [11].

It is worth taking a step back and thinking about the apparent dichotomy between rodent and large animal studies. Although the large animals previously described have been shown to develop ARONJ in some cases/experiments, it is nowhere near the incidence rate commonly found in rodent papers (in which anywhere from 50–100% of animals get ARONJ). As outlined in the section describing the advantages and disadvantages of large animal models, there are a number of potential explanations. As the field moves forward it will be important to understand the underlying mechanism to explain these findings. Most importantly however, it will be necessary to utilize both small and large animal models to make progress in the field of ARONJ.

5   Microvascular possibilities and limitations?

Treatment strategies for manifest ARONJ have been changing over recent years. While the first guidelines suggest a strictly conservative approach with antibiotics and mouth rinses [12], more recently, an early surgical approach with complete removal of the necrotic bone and safe primary wound closure is favored by a growing number of clinicians [5, 13–15]. However, even though patients can be released from open necrotic bone, functional reconstruction remains a challenge after the resection of the necrosis. In many patients, the retention of cover dentures is objectionable and endosteal implantation is regarded as hazard for the development of new ARONJ lesions. Bone augmentation after resection and healing of ARONJ seems to be one of the next major challenges.

Lesions from ARONJ emerge more frequently in the mandible, and large lesions can lead to pathological fractures. Especially when these lesions progress from the alveolar crest to the border of the mandible, they can be regarded as defect fractures. Treatment of the pathological fractures of patients undergoing BP treatment is still an unsolved issue [16].

Microvascular anastomosed bone transplants are usually preferred in areas with impaired wound healing. Several case reports refer that after resection of ARONJ, jaw continuity had been successfully reconstructed using fibula grafts [17]. Nevertheless, the donor site morbidity is considerably higher than in nonvascularized bone grafts.

Only a few studies have been published using microvascular bone transfer for mandible reconstruction [18]. After an anatomical study of the vascularization of the minipig's iliac crest, Schmelzeisen et al published several articles on the transplantation of vascularized iliac crest bone grafts to the mandible of Göttingen minipigs [19]. Although a constant vascular supply to the graft was restored in these animals, new bone formation was delayed, and the major part of the bone marrow was necrosed. The vascularized femoral flap has been the focus of a number of publications on reconstruction of mandibular defects in pigs and was shown to have less bone resorption than nonvascularized transplants [20]. Prefabricated vascularized bone grafts using recombinant osteogenic protein-1 have also been used in pigs. In dogs, the harvest of fibular bone grafts has been described and reconstruction of radiated mandibles with microvascular anastomosed composite rib grafts has been carried out successfully [21, 22].

Bone and fracture healing using microvascular bone transfer is thought to be one of the next steps in ARONJ large animal research, however, to the authors' best knowledge, due to the complex nature and high costs of large animal models, it is yet to have been conducted.

6 Conclusion

Antiresorptive drug-related osteonecrosis of the jaw can be reliably and reproducibly related in large animals. Due to the fact that the anatomy and bone physiology of large animals resemble their human counterparts more closely than small animals such as rodents, these larger animal models are very important in getting greater insight into the pathophysiology of this disease. Furthermore, improvement in ARONJ treatment and prophylactic measures continue to be investigated.

7 References

1. **Reinwald S, Burr D.** Review of nonprimate, large animal models for osteoporosis research. *J Bone Miner Res.* 2008 Sep; 23(9):1353–1368.
2. **Allen MR.** Animal models of medication-related osteonecrosis of the jaw. In: Otto S (ed). *Medication-Related Osteonecrosis of the Jaws.* Berlin Heidelberg: Springer; 2015:155–167.
3. **Allen MR, Burr DB.** The pathogenesis of bisphosphonate-related osteonecrosis of the jaw: so many hypotheses, so few data. *J Oral Maxillofac Surg.* 2009 May; 67(5 Suppl):S61–70.
4. **Pautke C, Kreutzer K, Weitz J, et al.** Bisphosphonate related osteonecrosis of the jaw: A minipig large animal model. *Bone.* 2012 Sep; 51(3):592–599.
5. **Voss PJ, Joshi Oshero J, Kovalova-Muller A, et al.** Surgical treatment of bisphosphonate-associated osteonecrosis of the jaw: technical report and follow up of 21 patients. *J Craniomaxillofac Surg.* 2012 Dec; 40(8):719–725.
6. **Allen MR, Kubek DJ, Burr DB, et al.** Compromised osseous healing of dental extraction sites in zoledronic acid-treated dogs. *Osteoporos Int.* 2011 Feb; 22(2):693–702.
7. **Voss PJ, Stoddart M, Ziebart T, et al.** Zoledronate induces osteonecrosis of the jaw in sheep. *J Craniomaxillofac Surg.* 2015 Sep; 43(7):1133–1138.
8. **Voss PJ, Stoddart MJ, Bernstein A, et al.** Zoledronate induces bisphosphonate-related osteonecrosis of the jaw in osteopenic sheep. *Clin Oral Investig.* 2016 Jan; 20(1):31–38.
9. **Allen MR.** Bisphosphonates and osteonecrosis of the jaw: moving from the bedside to the bench. *Cells Tissues Organs.* 2009; 189(1–4):289–294.
10. **Allen MR, Burr DB.** Mandible matrix necrosis in beagle dogs after 3 years of daily oral bisphosphonate treatment. *J Oral Maxillofac Surg.* 2008 May; 66(5):987–994.
11. **Allen MR, Chu TM, Ruggiero SL.** Absence of exposed bone following dental extraction in beagle dogs treated with 9 months of high-dose zoledronic acid combined with dexamethasone. *J Oral Maxillofac Surg.* 2013 Jun; 71(6):1017–1026.
12. **Marx RE, Sawatari Y, Fortin M, et al.** Bisphosphonate-induced exposed bone (osteonecrosis/osteopetrosis) of the jaws: risk factors, recognition, prevention, and treatment. *J Oral Maxillofac Surg.* 2005 Nov; 63(11):1567–1575.
13. **Pautke C.** Treatment of medication-related osteonecrosis of the jaw. In: Otto S (ed). *Medication-Related Osteonecrosis of the Jaws.* Berlin Heidelberg: Springer; 2015:79–92.
14. **Pautke C, Bauer F, Tischer T, et al.** Fluorescence-guided bone resection in bisphosphonate-associated osteonecrosis of the jaws. *J Oral Maxillofac Surg.* 2009 Mar; 67(3):471–476.
15. **Stockmann P, Vairaktaris E, Wehrhan F, et al.** Osteotomy and primary wound closure in bisphosphonate-associated osteonecrosis of the jaw: a prospective clinical study with 12 months follow-up. *Support Care Cancer.* 2010 Apr; 18(4):449–460.
16. **Otto S, Pautke C, Hafner S, et al.** Pathologic fractures in bisphosphonate-related osteonecrosis of the jaw-review of the literature and review of our own cases. *Craniomaxillofac Trauma Reconstr.* 2013 Sep; 6(3):147–154.

17. **Mucke T, Haarmann S, Wolff KD, et al.** Bisphosphonate related osteonecrosis of the jaws treated by surgical resection and immediate osseous microvascular reconstruction. *J Craniomaxillofac Surg.* 2009 Jul; 37(5):291–297.

18. **Carlson ER, Basile JD.** The role of surgical resection in the management of bisphosphonate-related osteonecrosis of the jaws. *J Oral Maxillofac Surg.* 2009 May; 67(5 Suppl):S85–95.

19. **Schmelzeisen R, Schon R.** Microvascular reanastomozed allogenous iliac crest transplants for the reconstruction of bony defects of the mandible in miniature pigs. *Int J Oral Maxillofac Surg.* 1998 Oct; 27(5):377–385.

20. **Benlidayi ME, Gaggl A, Buerger H, et al.** Comparison of vascularized osteoperiosteal femur flaps and nonvascularized femur grafts for reconstruction of mandibular defects: an experimental study. *J Oral Maxillofac Surg.* 2009 Jun; 67(6):1174–1183.

21. **Altobelli DE, Lorente CA, Handren JH, Jr.**, et al. Free and microvascular bone grafting in the irradiated dog mandible. *J Oral Maxillofac Surg.* 1987 Jan; 45(1):27–33.

22. **Shaffer JW, Field GA, Goldberg VM, et al.** A vascularized fibula model to study vascularized canine bone grafts. *Microsurgery.* 1984; 5(4):185–190.